The
Compassionate
Mind
Workbook

The Compassionate Mind Workbook

CHRIS IRONS and ELAINE BEAUMONT

ROBINSON

First published in Great Britain in 2017 by Robinson

10

A CIP catalogue record for this book
is available from the British Library.

ISBN: 978-1-47213-590-2

Typeset in Palatino by Initial Typesetting Services
Printed and bound in Great Britain by Bell & Bain

Papers used by Robinson are from well-managed forests and
other responsible sources.

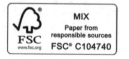

Robinson
An imprint of
Little, Brown Book Group
Carmelite House
50 Victoria Embankment
London EC4Y 0DZ

An Hachette UK Company
www.hachette.co.uk

www.littlebrown.co.uk

For Sue and Korina

Contents

Section VII
PUTTING OUR COMPASSIONATE MIND TO WORK WITH COMMON DIFFICULTIES

Section VIII
LOOKING FORWARD: SUSTAINING OUR COMPASSIONATE MIND

Acknowledgements

We would both like to thank our clients, past and present, who we have worked with over the years. Working alongside you, witnessing your courage and wisdom in the face of adversity, is a privilege and an honour.

We would like to express our heartfelt gratitude to Paul Gilbert, the team at The Compassionate Mind Foundation and colleagues and friends from the CFT community – Michelle Cree, Dennis Tirch, Mary Welford, Russell Kolts, Tobyn Bell, Charlie Heriot-Maitland, Deborah Lee, Kate Lucre, Gill Rayner, Jean Gilbert and many others. Your guidance while we wrote this book has been invaluable and we are very grateful for the support you have given to us throughout this process.

We would also like to acknowledge and thank Tobyn Bell, Charlie Heriot-Maitland, Tim LeBon, Sue Massey and Dennis Tirch for looking through drafts and for giving helpful direction and suggestions for this book. A special thank you to Korina Ioannou for all your hard work, help and wisdom – this book wouldn't be what it is without your help.

Thank you also to Andrew McAleer, Jane Donovan and Rebecca Sheppard at Little, Brown for all your help, support and patience!

Elaine:

Thank you to my friends and colleagues, past and present, at the University of Salford – you continue to encourage, nurture, teach and inspire me. Thanks also to the students at the University of Salford who enthusiastically volunteered their time, giving feedback regarding many of the exercises in this book; teaching you is a pleasure.

Thank you to family and friends who have encouraged and supported me while writing this book, and to Sr Anne O'Shea, a remarkable woman who inspired me to work in the helping profession. Sadly she is no longer with us, but her light continues to shine.

Finally, thank you to Sue. Without your support, unfailing belief in me, compassion and good humour, this would not have been possible.

Chris:

A big thank you to my current and past colleagues who have assisted and supported me in my interest in Compassion Focused Therapy. Thank you to my family and friends for all your love, care and backing – it's a powerful thing to know that you have people behind you in this way.

A special thank you to Paul Gilbert. I don't get enough opportunities to say how appreciative I am of you mentoring, support and friendship.

Finally, a massive thank you to my wife, Korina. Words can't describe my appreciation of your love and encouragement. Thank you for allowing me to be this version of myself!

Introduction

Welcome to *The Compassionate Mind Workbook*. This book focuses on how developing compassion for ourselves and others can help us to navigate the ups, downs and struggles that are common in life. In the last twenty years there has been an increasing amount of research showing how practising compassion can change the way we think, feel and behave – and even how our bodies and brains work. It is easy for people to misunderstand compassion though – as something soft, fluffy, indulgent or even weak. In reality, compassion is one of the wisest and most courageous motivations we have! Think about it for a moment: it's often a compassionate motivation that leads to training to join the services of fire, sea and air; it's a compassionate motivation that leads us towards studying for many years to become part of a helping profession, such as a teacher, doctor or nurse. Indeed, any time we want to make a difference to somebody, to be helpful and supportive in times they are struggling, we are engaging our compassion motivation. If you take a moment to think about people who are known for being compassionate – maybe people like Jesus, Mahatma Gandhi or Nelson Mandela – these were not weak people but rather, people determined to bring a compassionate approach to the world. There is absolutely nothing weak, fluffy or soft about compassion; it is the most important of all our motives. The problem is that for many reasons we do not remember to work from this motivation, and instead act out of anger, hatred, fear, shame or even self-criticism and self-dislike.

Although we will return to this in more detail in Chapter 4, it may be helpful early on to clarify what compassion is, and what it isn't. As one of our clients said to one of us: 'The biggest problem with compassion is the word itself!' This turned out to be an important insight and one shared by other clients, therapists and people in general when it comes to thinking about developing compassion.

What's in a word?

Some of the difficulties with compassion relate to the word itself. When we introduce the idea of compassion to people and ask them to name the words they feel are associated with it, many describe a variety of positively directed terms, including care, kindness, warmth, patience, empathy and understanding. However, sometimes people name negatively associated words such as pity, weakness, indulgence, 'letting myself off the hook' and even 'wishy-washy'.

Think about the word 'compassion' – does it have any negative associations for you? What do you not like about it?

_____

_____

_____

Of course, if you do have some negatively loaded terms that pop up in your head, that's not your fault. However, it might make it difficult for you to practise becoming more compassionate with yourself or others if that's the case! So to start with we just want to let you know that for us, compassion is none of those negative terms.

In the approach we will take in this book, compassion is a 'sensitivity to suffering in self and others, with a commitment to alleviate and prevent it'. So based on this definition, compassion requires certain qualities of mind. First, we need to develop a preparedness to pay attention to things that are difficult without turning away, avoiding, switching off, or simply reaching for that bottle of wine. This means we develop the courage to turn towards our own and others' difficulties, not away from them. This book will explore how we develop the strength and courage that allows us to do this. Second, we need to develop wisdom in our desire to be caring and helpful; so unfortunately, good intention is not enough, we also need to develop a variety of skills that help us to work with our own and others' difficulties and distress. Here's an example: suppose you see somebody fall into a river. Because they look like they're drowning, *Baywatch* style, you run up to the edge of the water and dive in to save them. Certainly a compassionate thing to do, right? Well yes, but only if you can swim. If you can't, then sadly both of you are likely to drown, and this *wouldn't* have been a compassionate behaviour. Here's another example: if you wanted to be a doctor and help people, it would be important for you to pay attention to people's distress, pain and suffering, but you would also need to study for many years to acquire wisdom to know how best to do this. You have intuitive wisdom about how many things in life involve the development of skills and knowledge – if you want to be good at the guitar, or golf, or teaching, what do you have to do? So we all know that practice, and the acquisition of skills, are important in many areas of life.

It turns out that it's the same for compassion, and our minds. The more we understand our minds and in particular, the more we understand how to look after them and cultivate them, the happier we're likely to be. In our culture we teach many important subjects at school – maths, languages, science and so forth – but sadly, we don't learn about how our minds work, and the skills we need to practise to help create healthy and supportive relationships with ourselves and others. In fact, unfortunately, much of modern life – our schools, work-places and media – does the opposite; moving us into a competitive self-focus, with concerns about the need to succeed, worrying about not being good enough, attractive enough or talented enough. Research shows that we are increasingly dissatisfied with ourselves to the point where we can struggle with mental health problems like anxiety and depression. This is a tragedy of modern society, and for our minds and bodies.

However, let's imagine that you could develop the skills and learn to find ways to work with the difficulties we can face in life through focusing on your desire to be helpful, sup-portive, strong and insightful. Imagine that you could learn how to slow down and tune in to your inner wisdom to help yourself with whatever difficulties you face. If that appeals to you then you're reading the right book! This is what compassion training is all about, and why this book is for you. So if you're someone who becomes self-critical when you make mistakes; or someone who worries about lots of things, like what other people think about you or your performance at work; or if you find that you ruminate on problems, and the mistakes you feel you've made – imagine learning how to stand back, notice what's hap-pening in your mind, and being able to bring your compassionate courage and wisdom to the problem.

It might be that reading this you're thinking: 'That's not possible! I've always been a self-critical person/a worrier/someone who ruminates a lot.' Or you might also be thinking: 'But all of those things are important parts of who I am – I get through my difficulties by criticising myself/worrying/ruminating.' This book will help you to practise developing a different way to treat yourself and others when things are difficult. It builds on considerable research that has found that by practising compassion we may become less self-critical, anxious, angry and depressed, whilst experiencing greater well-being and relationship satisfaction. Some of the training exercises we're going to share (we'll refer to them as Compassionate Mind Training or 'CMT' exercises) with you have been developed over many hundreds of years in contemplative traditions. Others, however, have been developed from working with people who have a range of emotional difficulties, and were developed in a therapy called Compassion Focused Therapy (CFT). But you don't need to be in therapy, or even feel like you need to be, to benefit from the ideas and practices that we'll explore together in the coming chapters. All of us will experience suffering in life – setbacks, failures, rejections, painful feelings and emotions and sadly, ill health and death. It is because of this that learning to develop our compassionate minds is something we can benefit from.

So let's take a journey into how we can develop our compassionate minds, and in doing so, learn how to bring compassion in to our everyday lives and help us deal with the difficulties, setbacks and fears that can so easily capture us and cause us distress.

How is the book organised?

The approach we are going to take is partly derived from Compassion Focused Therapy (CFT). In this therapy we use a lot of mind training practice, such as learning to pay attention in certain ways, behavioural practices, ways of imagining things to stimulate our brains and bodies, and developing identity based around the qualities of compassion. This book brings these exercises and practices to you in a structured way allowing you to gain the benefit of compassionate mind training. We've split the book into the following sections:

Section I: Why we need compassion

In this section we're going to look at some of the most important things we need to know about how our human mind actually got to be the way it is. We will explore ideas about how it works, and how it is so easy for us to be carried away with anger, anxiety and self-doubt; why is it so easy for us to become tribal, hostile and aggressive to each other; and why it is so easy for us to struggle with a variety of mental health problems like depression, even though our material lives are much better than they were, say, five hundred years ago. We will learn that whilst having wonderful abilities, the human brain has a lot of built-in problems because of the way it has evolved. When we really understand this, we can then see that many of the difficulties we have with the way our minds work are not really our fault. However, this understanding doesn't lead to giving up; rather, it can inspire us to learn how to take responsibility for our minds by learning certain mind training practices.

Section II: Understanding compassion

In the second section of the book, we'll explore in more detail what we mean by compassion. We'll explore some of the qualities that are helpful in building a compassionate mind, and outline how compassion has three 'flows': the compassion you have for other people, being open to compassion from others, and compassion for yourself (self-compassion). We'll also take a look at some of the blocks and fears that can arise about compassion, and see how these can get in the way of developing our compassionate minds.

Section III: Building capacity: Developing the foundations for our compassionate mind

The third part of this book focuses on helping us to create the sound foundations for compassion. Just like building a house first needs time spent on laying firm foundation stones, it's helpful to consider a similar process for developing your compassionate mind. So in the chapters in this section, we'll look together at cultivating your attention and awareness skills through various mindfulness practices, before going on to introduce ways that you can develop your positive emotion systems, which have been found to be powerful ways of helping us to manage our distress in life.

Section IV: Developing our compassionate mind

In the chapters in this section we'll help you to develop your compassionate mind. This will involve learning about and then practising exercises that are key to CMT – such as 'compassionate self' – and which with practice, can help people to manage their difficulties in a different way.

Section V: Directing our compassionate mind: Compassion as flow

In these chapters we'll explore how compassion can come in three different flows: to others, from others, and to ourselves (self-compassion). Just like the three legs of a stool, we want each of these 'flows' to be firm and steady, and we'll outline different ways in which we can practise and strengthen our ability to do this.

Section VI: Developing the skills of our compassionate mind

In this section of the book, we'll help you to focus your developing 'compassionate mind' in some important ways – in shaping your motivation, attention, thinking, feelings and behaviour. In each of these areas we'll help you to practise ways to guide your compassionate mind in skilful ways, which have been shown to help people manage the difficulties and distress in their life.

Section VII: Putting our compassionate mind to work with common difficulties

Now that you've got a firm grounding in the attributes and skills of your compassionate mind, we'll focus on how you can apply these skills to help with the common difficulties that many of us struggle with – difficulties with self-criticism, and struggles to manage our emotions.

Section VIII: Looking forward: Sustaining our compassionate mind

In the final section, and in fact the final chapter of this book, we'll spend time considering how to sustain the work you've done to develop your compassionate mind. We'll explore common ways that people can get side-tracked or experience setbacks, and find ways to plan for these (as best as we can) whilst focusing on the intention to support yourself as you move forward.

How to use this book

This book has been designed as a step-by-step guide to helping you develop your compassionate mind. As we've just highlighted, each section of this book contains a number of chapters to help you develop your understanding of, and skills to manage, the difficulties and distress you experience in life and to increase your wellbeing. We have set out each chapter so that there are opportunities for personal reflection on what you've been learning, and opportunities to learn and practise a variety of skills.

Practise

As you proceed through the book, try and make a commitment to practise the techniques and skills in each chapter. It's important to give yourself the time to practise the exercises in each chapter, even if some of them are tricky or you feel the urge to move on to the next exercise or chapter. Like learning most new skills, this takes a bit of practice and at times, patience – but over time will become easier.

The book aims to help you train your mind to compassionately respond to suffering and to bring balance to your life. In some of the chapters we have a helpful hints section and a common difficulties section to help you along the way. Go at your own pace, but remember the idea of 'small steps'; so just as we learn to swim in the shallow end of the pool (rather than the middle of an ocean during a storm!), the same applies here. Take your time and gradually build up your confidence through practising as often as you can. If you find yourself racing through exercises without really tuning in and connecting with them, then it might be helpful to take a pause, and return to trying them out at a later time in the day or week.

Be kind to yourself

Try to remember to be kind to yourself as you work through each chapter. This is especially the case if you are finding something difficult or have a setback – we all have setbacks and although we can learn from them, they can still be painful experiences. Sometimes here it can be helpful to start with reminding ourselves of our intention and focusing on our desire to learn how to be more caring and compassionate to ourselves, including in the moments we struggle.

Case examples

To help bring some of the ideas and practices of this book alive, we have used a number of case examples throughout the book. These are mostly amalgamations of real people and our personal experiences. All names and personal details have been changed to protect anonymity.

Section I

WHY WE NEED COMPASSION

The first section of the workbook outlines the reasons why developing compassion for ourselves and others may be helpful. We will explore three compassionate insights in the following chapters:

- That our minds have evolved in a way that makes them quite 'tricky' and naturally vulnerable to getting caught up in thinking-feeling loops that can drive distress

- That we are shaped by experiences that we have little control over

- That we have three core emotion systems that evolved to serve important functions, but which can easily get out of balance.

We'll also explore how we can integrate these ideas into helping you to understand yourself, and some of the difficulties you face.

1 We have tricky brains

'The mind is its own place, and in itself can make a Heaven of Hell, a Hell of Heaven.'

– John Milton, Paradise Lost, Book I

Life can be hard, can't it? Sometimes this is because of what's happening in *our* lives: work, family or relationship stress, bad memories from the past or maybe a serious illness we're suffering from. Other times it can be linked to the reality of looking out around us to the suffering in the world: wars, poverty, natural disasters and famines – or the realisation that at some stage, we are all going to die. These are not things we like to focus on, and for the most part not useful to do for too long. But sometimes it's important for us to acknowledge the reality of life and find a way we can work with this, rather than ignoring it, fighting it off or trying to block it out of our minds. This is where compassion comes in because it provides the grounding of a wise and courageous base for us to work with life's realities.

One of the cornerstones of compassion is wisdom. This means that to develop your compassionate mind, acquiring the wisdom in understanding how and why we suffer may be an important step in helping ourselves to relieve this. We can look for the causes of suffering in different places. For example, falling off your bike and breaking your arm would be causes of suffering (pain). But we can also look behind the scenes to help us with this: the reason we feel physical pain is because evolution has built bodies capable of feeling physical pain, so as to signal us to potential dangers and the need to care for our body if we have been hurt in some way (for example, cleaning out a wound, or resting when you have a sprained ankle). So an important starting point in understanding our minds is to learn about how they work; how they got to be the way they are. Compassionate Mind Training (CMT) highlights how some of the problems that we experience in life are linked to how our mind evolved.

It turns out that the process of evolution has actually left our brains in a bit of a mess! We refer to this as how we all have 'tricky brains'. Our brains are capable of amazing things, and they give rise to wonderful abilities such as the ability to think, imagine, plan and reflect.

These in turn gave rise to some of the great accomplishments of our species: the writings of Shakespeare, Hemingway and Austen; the art of Michelangelo and Picasso, the music of Beethoven and Mozart. It's led to amazing medical advancements – antibiotics, medicines and operations – that have saved the lives of millions. Science has opened our eyes to the building blocks of ourselves and the universe – and helped to land people on the moon. Unfortunately, these same abilities for thinking, reasoning, and imagining also have a dark side. We have an inexhaustible way of bringing pain to others. We have invented weapons of mass destruction and polluted our planet. And these same abilities can also drive much of our own distress through self-criticism, worry and rumination.

A useful albeit simplified way of understanding the human brain is to think about old and new parts. There are parts of our brains that are very ancient (over 200 million years old) which we share with many other species of animals (e.g. reptiles and mammals) – and a part of our mind that is more recently evolved, and that has some uniquely 'human' functions. We refer to these as our 'old brain' and our 'new brain'.

Our old brain: just like our bodies, our brain is the product of hundreds of millions of years of evolution. Some of its oldest structures appear to function in a way that helps us – and other animals who share similar brain structures – to navigate many of the dangers in the world in a safe way, and be motivated to pursue resources that may be beneficial for survival and reproduction.

Scientists sometimes talk about how these brain structures originated in the reptiles – and this part of the brain is often referred to as the 'reptilian brain'. In fact, they sometimes joke that the function of this old part of the brain is linked to the four Fs: feeding, fighting, fleeing and … having sex! These are all motives that you will see reptiles engage in, but because our brains have retained similar structures, they are also important motives for us as well. Following after the reptiles, about 200 million years ago mammals emerged into the world. Similar to the reptiles, mammals also have an interest in the four Fs, but have a greater interest in, and ways of caring for, their offspring. They are also more orientated to and motivated to engage in bonding, social communication, play and affection. This part of the brain is sometimes referred to as the mammalian brain, or limbic system, and is likely to play an important role in the functioning of basic emotions like anxiety, anger, sadness and joy, which evolved to help animals engage with their motives and, ultimately, survive and prosper.

Summary: so we have explored how we have an 'old' part of our brains with a range of functions: motives, emotions and basic defensive behaviours that we share with other animals in the world that were shaped by evolution to facilitate survival and reproduction. These include:

• Basic motives such as harm-avoidance (survival), seeking of food, sexual opportunities and status; for attachment and caring for offspring

• Defensive behaviours such as fight, flight, freeze, submission and clinging

• Basic emotions such as anger, anxiety, disgust, sadness and joy.

> *Claire's old brain example:* Claire was having big problems at work. Her boss was often very critical, harsh and dismissive, and at times, emotionally abusive. To make matters worse, her colleagues were very competitive and unsupportive. When she thought about how this was impacting on her old brain, she recognised that in this environment, she was left feeling very anxious (almost continually), and had an urge to 'flee' and avoid being in the office. She also recognised that she didn't do this partly because it was important to her that she was successful and earned 'good money', so often had to behave in a very submissive, non-challenging way with colleagues.

Self-reflection: Exploring your old brain

Can you think of common times – or types of situations – where your old brain has been triggered?

Which old brain emotion did this situation trigger for you?

What motivation or behaviours tend to come with this? What do you want to do when this old brain emotion is triggered?

_____

_____

However, as a species we've also developed a set of more recently evolved ('new') competencies.

Our new brain 'human' abilities: Around two million years ago, our distant primate ancestors started to develop increasingly complex, sophisticated and 'intelligent' thinking abilities. This part of our brain is linked to part of the brain called the prefrontal cortex, and gave rise to wonderful new abilities in the world. These include:

- Our ability to *imagine* things. We have an amazing ability to create images in our minds that may or may not be real, but help us in many areas of life. Whether an artist or author, architect or actor, our capacity to create images is essential in all of these careers. We also use our imagination to navigate our social relationships. Think about the last time you had to buy a present for a friend, or planned a surprise for someone you care for. It's likely your capacity to imagine was central to this.

- We can *consider the future*: our new brain competencies allow us to cast our mind forward to the future and consider potential outcomes. We can plan for things that may or may not happen, whether that is later today, next week, next year or in ten years' time.

- We can *think about our thinking*. This is sometimes referred to as 'metacognition', and reflects how our new brain abilities can lead to a capacity to monitor our own minds, and form beliefs about our own minds, thoughts and feelings.

- We can reflect on things in the *past*: it's not just the future that we can contemplate; we can transport our minds back in time and ruminate over things that have happened – and things that we have done and have been done to us – in the past.

Although two million years sounds like an awfully long time, in evolutionary terms it is quite a recent development (the earliest basic life forms on earth are estimated to have evolved around four billion years ago!), so we therefore refer to these new brain abilities or functions. As we touched on above, these new brain abilities have allowed humans to do wonderful things – to write great works of poetry and fiction, to paint, draw and sculpt, and more recently, to develop an understanding of nature, science and technology. We have developed cures for a myriad of illnesses, developed technology to scan inside our bodies, and sent men and women into space. However, as you might be able to tell, there is a 'but' to this.

Old and new 'loops' – a mind that can turn in on itself

Although we are simplifying complex brain processes here, we know that our new competencies for thinking, imagining, ruminating, worrying and self-awareness can interact well with our old brain motives, emotions and behaviours, and can sit alongside each other in a coordinated, helpful way (this is depicted in Figure 1.1 below).

Figure 1.1 Interacting old and new brain functions

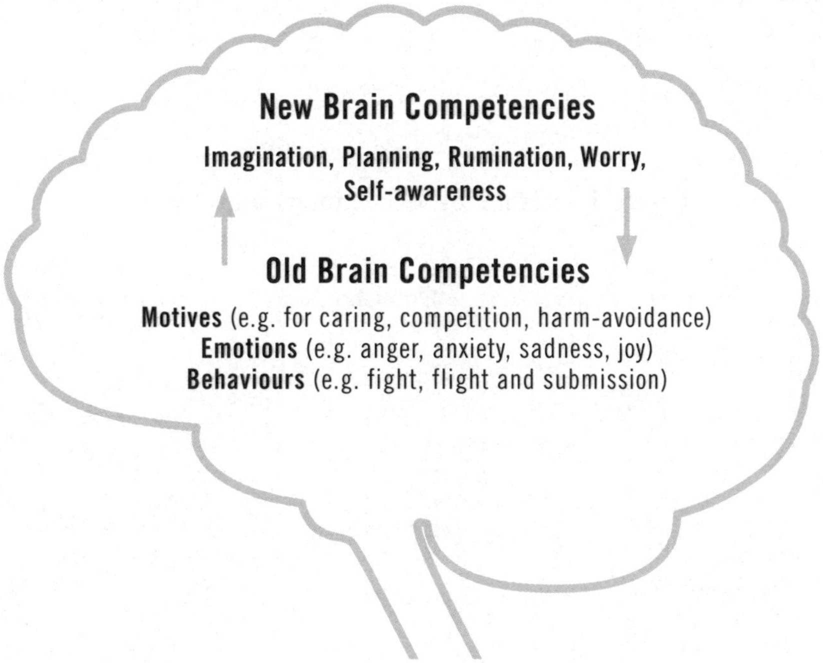

New Brain Competencies

Imagination, Planning, Rumination, Worry, Self-awareness

Old Brain Competencies

Motives (e.g. for caring, competition, harm-avoidance)
Emotions (e.g. anger, anxiety, sadness, joy)
Behaviours (e.g. fight, flight and submission)

However, at times these different new and old functions can get caught up in unhelpful 'loops'. Our mind can turn in on itself in a way that can lead to 'glitches', which in turn can drive some of the distress and difficulties we experience in life.

Here are some examples:

Example 1: John was in bed, feeling relaxed after a long day at work. Just as he was about to fall asleep, a thought popped into his mind: 'Did I remember to lock the office properly?' Suddenly, his sleepiness disappeared, and he began to feel a little tension and anxiety in his stomach. Two hours later he was still awake, struggling with insomnia, tense and frustrated. His mind was going round in circles, not just about the unlocked office door, but images of all the computers and company secrets missing in the morning! As this feeling of anxiety continued, a new set of thoughts emerged: 'Why am I so forgetful – maybe there's something wrong with me' which continued to leave him feeling anxious and tense. Figure 1.2 shows John's loops drawn out.

Figure 1.2: Some of John's loops drawn out

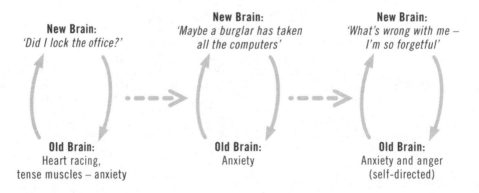

New Brain:
'Did I lock the office?'

New Brain:
'Maybe a burglar has taken all the computers'

New Brain:
'What's wrong with me – I'm so forgetful'

Old Brain:
Heart racing, tense muscles – anxiety

Old Brain:
Anxiety

Old Brain:
Anxiety and anger (self-directed)

Example 2: Naz was checking Facebook when she saw a picture of a number of close friends having – by the looks on their faces – a great time at a party of another friend. Moreover, the comment next to the picture read: 'All the best friends together – greatest party ever!' Just seeing the picture and reading the comment, Naz began to feel tense and anxious, and a thought entered her mind: 'They're having such a great time – how come I didn't get invited?' and 'Maybe I didn't get invited because I didn't send Sarah a birthday card.' These thoughts and feelings started to churn through her mind, leaving her feeling low in mood and sad, and led her to reflect on herself: 'I'm such a crap friend, it's my fault I didn't get invited.' After a while of feeling like this, a new thought entered her mind: 'Sarah knew why I didn't send her a card; she said she understood so this is her fault.' Naz noticed that she started to feel quite angry at Sarah, but also her other friends, and decided to send a text message to tell them what she thought of them all for being such bad, uncaring people. Figure 1.3 shows Naz's loops drawn out.

Figure 1.3: Some of Naz's loops drawn out

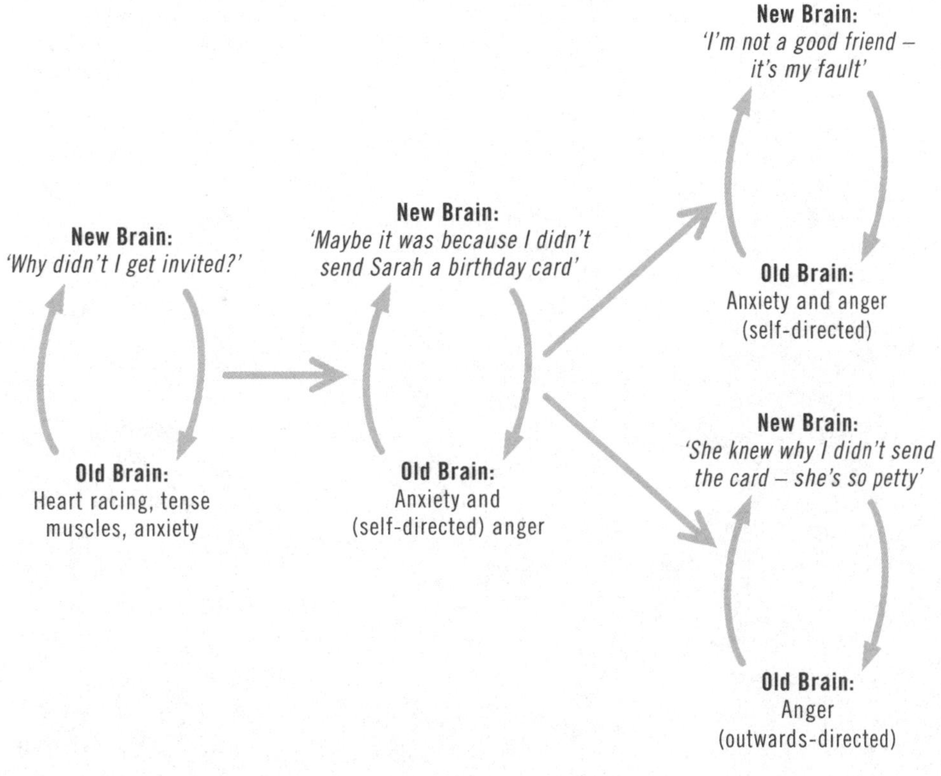

New Brain:
'Why didn't I get invited?'

Old Brain:
Heart racing, tense
muscles, anxiety

New Brain:
*'Maybe it was because I didn't
send Sarah a birthday card'*

Old Brain:
Anxiety and
(self-directed) anger

New Brain:
*'I'm not a good friend –
it's my fault'*

Old Brain:
Anxiety and anger
(self-directed)

New Brain:
*'She knew why I didn't send
the card – she's so petty'*

Old Brain:
Anger
(outwards-directed)

Example 3: Stephanie had a big presentation coming up at work, where she would have to talk to a large audience, many of them managers and executives in her company. The presentation was on a topic that was new to her (she had just moved jobs to a new department), and a lot rested on her doing a good job. Just the thought of presenting was making her feel anxious, and she began to get persistent worries running through her mind: 'What if I freeze and forget what to say?', 'What if they ask me questions that I can't answer?'. These thoughts often led her to get caught up with feeling more anxious, and sometimes she started to fantasise and plan for how she could get out of giving the talk: 'If I start coughing and saying I've got a headache in the week leading up, maybe I can call in sick.' Unfortunately, this just added to her feelings of anxiety, and made it harder to concentrate on preparing for the talk. This also triggered a series of more self-critical thoughts, which in turn triggered familiar feelings of self-directed anger, disgust and a sense of inferiority. Figure 1.4 shows Stephanie's loops drawn out.

Figure 1.4: Some of Stephanie's loops drawn out

New Brain:
'Maybe I can avoid doing it by pretending to be ill'

New Brain:
'I'm going to mess the presentation up'

New Brain:
'People will ask me questions I can't answer'

Old Brain:
Anxiety and avoidance

Old Brain:
Tense, anxious

Old Brain:
Anxiety

New Brain:
'I'm so pathetic and weak in comparison to others'

Old Brain:
Anger and disgust
(self-directed), inferiority

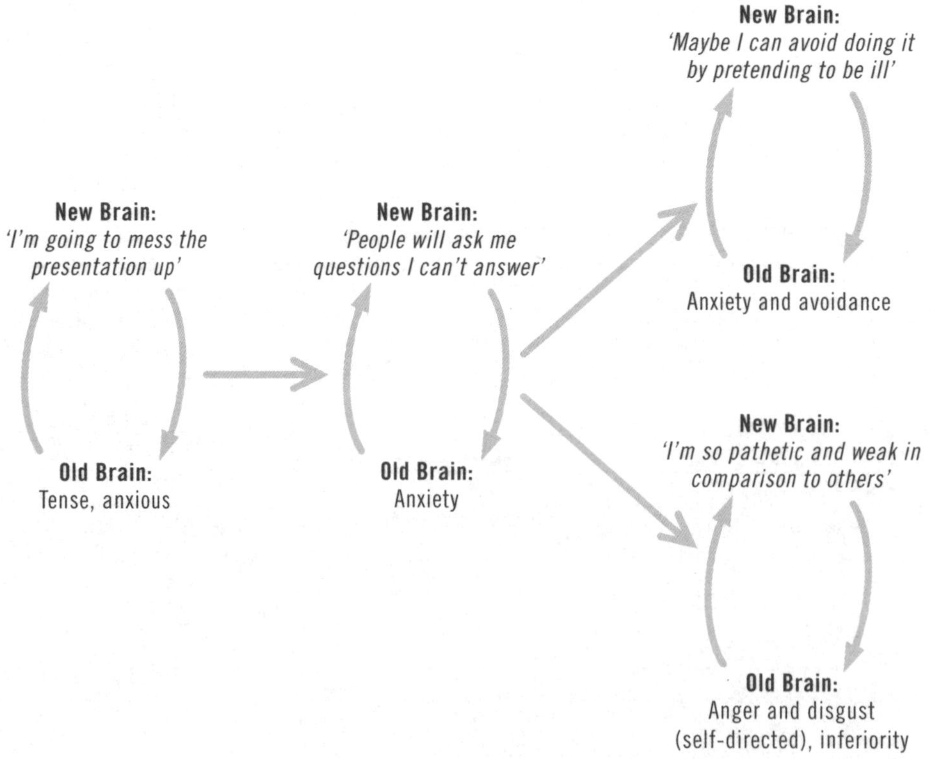

Worksheet 1.1: Personal example of my thinking loops

Given the above examples, it may be helpful to think about the type of 'loops in the mind' you experience. See if you can outline your own, specific loops below. It may help to start with thinking about a recent situation that might have triggered your loops. From this, see if you can begin to outline – like with the examples of John, Naz and Stephanie – loops you have between new brain competencies (e.g. thinking, worrying, imagining) and old brain emotions or behaviours (e.g. anger, anxiety, avoidance, aggression).

New Brain Competencies

(worries, ruminations, self-criticism)

_____

_____

_____

_____

_____

_____

Old Brain Competencies

(emotions, defensive behaviours)

_____

_____

_____

_____

_____

_____

What have you learnt about the loops between your new and old brain competencies?

_____

How often do you experience these types of loops?

_____

How do these loops affect your confidence, wellbeing or mood?

_____

A uniquely human problem?

As far as we know, these tricky 'loops in the mind' that can drive a lot of our distress are an exclusively human problem; other animals are unlikely to encounter these types of difficulties. For example, we don't think Spot the dog struggles at night with insomnia and anxiety, worrying about how he's put on some weight recently, and that the other local dogs won't find him attractive anymore! And he probably doesn't ruminate and beat himself up over his performance catching the Frisbee in the park the previous weekend. We don't think Moggy the cat gets caught up worrying about paying the bills, or ruminating about an argument she had the previous day either!

Here's another example that elaborates on this point. Imagine a zebra happily munching away on grass in the African savannah. Suddenly, it hears the breaking of twigs, and looks up to see a lion approaching. As zebras tend to do when they see lions approaching (outside of popular animated films, that is!), it stops eating and runs away (a basic old brain flight behaviour linked to the motive for self-preservation). Let's say that on this occasion our zebra is a quick runner, and manages to escape to live another day. What do you think the zebra will go back to doing relatively quickly after the threat of the lion has passed? That's right, it will probably return to eating grass again. So, once the external threat of the lion is gone, it calms down relatively quickly and returns to normal daily routines.

However, let's switch the example a bit. Imagine that you're sitting outside at a café, enjoying reading the paper and eating a tasty sandwich. As you turn the page over and look up, you notice a lion approaching the café (let's not worry too much how or why the lion got there!). Like the zebra, upon seeing the lion you also quickly get into old brain emotions (anxiety) and behaviours (running away). Imagine that like our friend the zebra, you managed to escape the lion by running into a building and locking the door behind you. Now that you're safe and away from the lion, would one of the first things you do involve finding the leftovers of that tasty sandwich you were eating?! If not, why not? Well, it turns out that us humans are able to do something that zebras can't – we can maintain a threat stimulus without the actual threat being there because we have new brain abilities that bring the stimulus inside our head. Through our new brain competencies of *imagination* (for example, picturing being eaten alive), *anticipation* (I wonder if the lion is still out there? And maybe it has friends) and *planning* (how am I going to be safe when I leave this building?) we can re-trigger our old brain capacity for emotions (anxiety) and protective behaviours (flight; shut down). In turn, this anxiety is likely to keep your attention, thinking and imagination focused upon the threat of the lion.

How can compassion help?

Earlier in this chapter, we mentioned that a key component of compassion is wisdom. One way that we can bring wisdom to the reality of our 'tricky brains' is to recognise that this is the case; to be open to the fact that our minds are often tricky and quite chaotic, but also to realise that this is *not our fault*. This can seem like a strange concept at first, but it turns out to be an important one in Compassionate Mind Training (CMT). Unfortunately, rather than supporting ourselves with our struggles in life, we can instead invalidate our own experiences or blame ourselves for them. We can tell ourselves that we *shouldn't* feel or think in a certain way – 'I should know better than to feel like this, it's my fault really and if only I just tried harder.' But it can be helpful to look at this from a different angle: although this can cause us distress and pain at times, *we did not choose* to have brains that have these different types of abilities for emotions and complex thinking. We did not choose to have a brain that could get caught up in loops.

If you think about it, how often do you wake up in the morning and think: 'I know what I'm going to do today, I'm going to start focusing my new brain competencies on all the things that are wrong with me in life, and that will then start to stimulate my old brain emotions of anxiety and sadness and de-motivate me...!' Probably not. Just as John, Naz and Stephanie didn't in their examples above. For most of us, of course, we just find that our mind starts working like this on its own, and at some stage we then become aware of it. But sadly, many of us blame ourselves for this, and this is why learning about how our brain has evolved can be *deshaming*. We can learn to realise that our mind seems to make lots of choices about what to focus on without much conscious input from us, the person who is supposed to be in charge.

So this is why in CMT we emphasise that we have *very* tricky brains, which naturally get caught up in thinking-feeling loops. This is not your fault – in fact, it's no one's fault. But whilst it may not be our fault that this happens, our compassionate wisdom helps us to take responsibility to learn what to do with them so that we don't suffer the consequences of these in a needless way. Although we will explore these in more detail in Chapters 8, 18 and 19, have a look at Box 1.1 overleaf for some ways that will help you to manage the loops in your mind.

Box 1.1: Some tips to help with the loops in your mind

Tips – initial steps to help with the loops in your mind

Although we do not choose to have these loops, we can do something about them. Here are some suggestions, which we will return to in later chapters.

- It can be helpful to become aware of the loops in your mind – if we notice them, then we might be able to do something about them. To do this, it can be helpful to learn more about the loops you experience. For example, for a week, at the end of each day take five minutes to write down the type of loops you got into that day. Or alternatively, using a notebook or your mobile phone, take regular notes throughout the day of the type of thinking-feeling loops you get into.

- If you find it hard to remember the type of loops you get into, set a reminder on your phone or computer to go off at regular intervals throughout the day. When this happens, take a moment to note down if you had just been experiencing any loops between your new and old brain competencies.

- Once we notice the loops, try to remember that these are perfectly normal and something that we all experience – there isn't anything wrong with you for having them.

- It can be helpful to find ways to notice that we are caught up in a loop, and practise ways of 'stepping out' of these. It could be that this is by re-directing your attention to something that is happening in the 'here and now' (for example, if I'm able to focus my mind on something that is happening right now, such as the sensation of my breathing, or the beautiful flowers and plants in my garden) this may slow or disrupt the loops. So rather than my attention being 'fully' caught in the loops, I am instead focusing on something neutral or pleasant instead. We will return to this idea when we practise attention and mindfulness training in Chapter 8.

- We can learn to hold the loops between thinking and feeling more 'loosely' in attention, so that we are aware of them but not feel that we have to fight or ignore them, push them out of mind or surrender to them. Instead, we can notice and observe these as just another 'product' of our minds that we did not choose to have. This can help us to move towards acceptance, which in and of itself can help them to soften and calm down. We will return to this in Chapter 8.

- We can learn to create a different pattern or 'loop' in our mind, one centred around compassionate intentions, thoughts and feelings. When we are connected to our compassionate minds, we trigger a different type of physiology in our brains and bodies than the (often) stress-based ones we've been exploring in this chapter. We will explore how we can practise this in Section III, and Chapters 9 and 10.

Chapter summary

We have covered a lot of ground in this first chapter. As we will at the end of each chapter, we have provided a summary of what we've explored in this chapter in the table below. Please take your time to make a few notes on your own reflections about what you've learned as well.

What we have learnt together	My personal reflections on the chapter
1. Our brain evolved in such a way that it has inbuilt glitches – it can get caught up in new brain-old brain loops and this, by its nature, can be very 'tricky'. 2. That as far as we know, other animals don't struggle with these types of difficulties. 3. That it's not our fault that we struggle with this – but that there are a number of things we can do to begin to help ourselves with this (e.g. noticing the types of loops we typically get caught in; to step back from blaming ourselves for this).	

2 We are shaped by our experiences

'We do not "come in" to the world, we come *out* of it.'

– Alan Watts, The Book on the Taboo Against Knowing Who You Are (1966)

Many of us intuitively know that the environments we grow up in have a very major impact on the person we become. Take language, for example. If you're raised in the UK or USA, it's likely that you'll speak English fluently. But if you're raised in Italy or Japan, it's far less likely you'll speak English, and far more likely you'll be fluent in Italian or Japanese. Religion is another example; statistically, you're far, far more likely to identify as Christian if you grow up in a Christian country, and Muslim if you grow up in a Muslim country. But it's not just at the level of language or belief that our environments influence us. Science is now helping us to understand that our environments shape our biology, our physiology; that different experiences in life shape the way our brains develop; and that even the way our genes express themselves can be affected by the environments in which we develop.

Although we like to think of ourselves as a particular kind of person, in fact we are simply one version – one version of many possible selves. Here's an example to consider. Although you don't know our backgrounds, imagine that as the people writing this book, rather than the experiences that have shaped and influenced us (our upbringing, parents, friends and so forth), we were instead abducted from the hospital at three days old by people who are the head of a violent drug gang. Imagine that we had been raised by these people and that as children and adolescents we had witnessed (and received) a lot of maltreatment, aggression and violence, and very little affection, support or encouragement. If this had been the case, how likely do you think it is that we'd both be therapists today, writing a book about compassion? If those had been our experiences, can you imagine what we might be like as people today? Maybe we would be struggling with anger and aggression, or alternatively, anxiety and non-assertiveness? Perhaps we would struggle to form close relationships, be addicted to drugs, or even be in prison. Although we cannot say for sure, what we can say is that we would be a different kind of person, with different personalities and even slightly different biology (genes, brain structure and so forth).

We can explore this idea through the example of Sarah in Figure 2.1 below. Take time to read through both scenarios – one that she did go through in life (Scenario 1), and an alternative set of life experiences (Scenario 2). Try to hold in mind how these different experiences might have shaped her as a person in different ways.

Figure 2.1: Sarah's life scenarios example

Scenario 1	Scenario 2
Sarah initially lived in a nice part of town, but after her dad died (he was serving in the army), her mum struggled to make ends meet. Aged seven, her family moved to a housing estate in a less affluent part of town, where many of the houses had broken windows and boarded-up doors. At times, there was not enough money to pay for food, heating or new clothes. Her mum was often tired from working two jobs, and at times could become very angry, critical and physically abusive. There was never any discussion about her dad's death, and Sarah often heard her mum crying late at night when she was in bed.	Sarah grew up in a nice part of town. Although not big, her house was clean, warm and tidy, and her family always ate dinner together every night. Although her dad was often away with work when she was young, when she was seven he left the army and trained to be a paramedic, working at the local hospital. Her parents both had well-paying, successful jobs, and took Sarah on regular holidays and outings. Although they would tell her off at times, she knew they loved her very much, and showed her a lot of affection, kindness and support.
Sarah attended a school that was put into special measures for poor academic achievement and unfortunately, she was bullied for not having 'trendy' clothes and shoes. Outside of school, she found it difficult to make friends, and often spent evenings and weekends in her bedroom on her own.	Sarah went to a good school, where she was encouraged to work hard, try out different subjects, hobbies and activities. She developed lots of good friends at school, and found it easy to turn to people when she needed help and support, but was also happy spending time on her own. Outside of school, she participated in lots of different activities, and found making friends very easy.

How did you feel reading through the scenarios above? Were you able to imagine how Sarah might be a different person if she'd had these different upbringings? Maybe you can imagine how, if you had been raised in either of these situations, there would be a different version of *you* in the world today.

Here's another short exercise you could try: consider how you might be different as a person today if you had been raised by your next-door neighbours, rather than in your house. Maybe spend thirty seconds or so imagining this. If this had been the case, how might you be different in terms of your personality, interests, politics and religion or the way you see yourself/other people?

Self-reflection: How might you be different today had you been raised by your neighbours?

_____

_____

_____

_____

Of course, we will never know for sure how these different scenarios would have influenced us, but what we do know is that the version of you that is reading this now is dependent upon the experiences that *you've* had. Change those experiences and you'd be a different person – there would be a *different version* of you in the world.

These examples can help us recognise that much of who we are today was shaped *for us*, and not *by us*. What we mean by this is that the person that you are right now reading this – and the people we are writing this – were highly influenced by events and experiences that have happened in our lives, many of which we had little or no control over. It can be tricky at times to hold onto these insights, and instead, many of us blame ourselves for the type of person we are – anxious, unconfident, angry, full of shame – which makes it less likely that we can do something about bringing change to our difficulties.

We can also see how our environment and experiences can have relevance for thinking about our future. Let's imagine for a moment Paul's situation.

Example: Paul has had a good life on the whole – caring parents, good experiences at school, a successful career and recently, he married his long-time partner, Andrew. Paul is a confident, outgoing person who enjoys going out, meeting people and having fun. One night when walking home from having a meal with a friend from work, he is mugged and beaten quite seriously. Paul is kept in hospital for a few days because of his injuries, and is then allowed to return home. So, following this horrible experience, do you think Paul will be exactly the same version of himself now? If not, how might you imagine the version of Paul changing – even in a small way? Maybe we could imagine him becoming a little more anxious leaving his home? Wary about travelling on his own? Less likely to trust people that he doesn't know? How might his relationship with Andrew change? Of course we can't know for sure, as we can respond in very different ways to this situation; however, what is likely is that it might bring a change to the *version of Paul* that was in the world before this incident.

How can compassion help with this?

Of course, it's not just negative experiences that affect the version of us in the world. There is a growing scientific literature showing that certain types of positive experiences in life can have knock-on, positive impacts upon us. For example, having people in our lives who support and care for us, feeling secure and safe, or learning new and more caring and helpful ways of thinking and treating ourselves can also bring about a change to the version of us here today. This is where Compassionate Mind Training (CMT), and this book, can play a role.

We're not suggesting that by developing compassion, we can change our past, or the experiences we've had in life. Nor is it just about trying to make us all 'think' positively about things. However, what we can all do is spend time practising ways to bring a slightly different version of ourselves into the world, a version that (surprise, surprise!) has a more compassionate, caring, understanding and confident way of dealing with the problems we can face in life. As the famous psychologist Carl Jung said, 'We meet ourselves time and again in a thousand disguises on the path of life.' It might be that through our life circumstances – many of which we have had little control or influence on – we 'meet' versions of ourselves that we are less happy with: versions that are lacking in confidence, or struggle to engage in things (relationships, hobbies, jobs) that might bring happiness or joy. Or we might meet versions that bring with them much distress and suffering: versions that are trapped with having experienced, and maybe re-experiencing, terrible traumas or abuses. Or versions laden with shame, self-hatred and anger. If these are the versions that we've met in life, maybe that you are currently 'with' as you're reading this book, then it might be that this is where compassion can help you – to become aware of, and practise, new versions of ourselves that might be more helpful and healthy for us.

Chapter summary

In this chapter we've started to explore how our social circumstances and experiences in life shape us as people. In Chapter 4 we look specifically at the factors that have shaped you.

What we have learnt together	My personal reflections on the chapter
1. We are shaped by our social experiences – many of which we have little control over. 2. That we are only one version of a potentially limitless number of versions of ourself; if we'd had different experiences in the past, we would likely be a different person today. 3. There is the possibility for different versions of us to exist in the world in the future – one way of bringing change is through developing your compassionate mind.	

3 Understanding our emotions

'Let's not forget that the little emotions are the great captains of our lives and we obey them without realising it.'

– *Vincent Van Gogh*

As we've explored so far, not only can life be hard, but our minds are vulnerable to getting caught up in a type of thinking-feeling loop that can drive a lot of our distress. Central to so much of this is emotion. Emotions are crucial in our lives; they provide the colour, richness and texture to our experiences. They also play an important role in providing us with feedback on how we are doing in life, guiding us towards things that are important and away from things that may be harmful.

There are many ways of exploring our emotions, and one that we will focus on here is how they can be grouped together based on their function – that is, what they help us to do. It's likely you already know this yourself. For example, if you're threatened in some way you might experience feelings of fear or anxiety. Or maybe, if this threat is in the form of being unfairly treated or blocked from doing something, you might experience anger and frustration. We often refer to these as 'threat emotions'. In contrast, if you're achieving things you might have pleasant emotions such as joy, excitement and happiness. We tend to describe these as positive emotions as they are associated with pleasurable feelings. However, we can also have positive emotions that are calming and soothing. For example, feeling relaxed, peaceful and contented. These emotions are most likely to be present *when we feel safe* and cared for.

Scientists have many theories about how many emotion 'systems' we have, but for the purposes of Compassionate Mind Training (CMT) and this workbook, we simplify this and suggest we all have three major emotion systems. These systems are depicted in Figure 3.1 overleaf, and this model is often referred to as the 'three-circle model' or the 'three-system model'. This model suggests that evolution has shaped our emotions to have different functions, all of which have been helpful in facilitating our chances for survival and reproduction and ultimately, passing on our genes. The three major emotion systems are referred to as *threat, drive* and *soothing* for short:

1. The threat system, with emotions of anger, fear and disgust, functions to help us identify and respond to threats in the world.

2. The drive system, linked to emotions of excitement and joy, motivates us to move towards resources and goals that might be helpful to us.

3. The soothing system, linked to feelings like contentment, calmness and safety, helps us to engage in periods of rest and peacefulness when we are not threatened or trying to achieve things. This system also orientates us to give and receive care from others.

Figure 3.1: The Three-System Model of Emotion

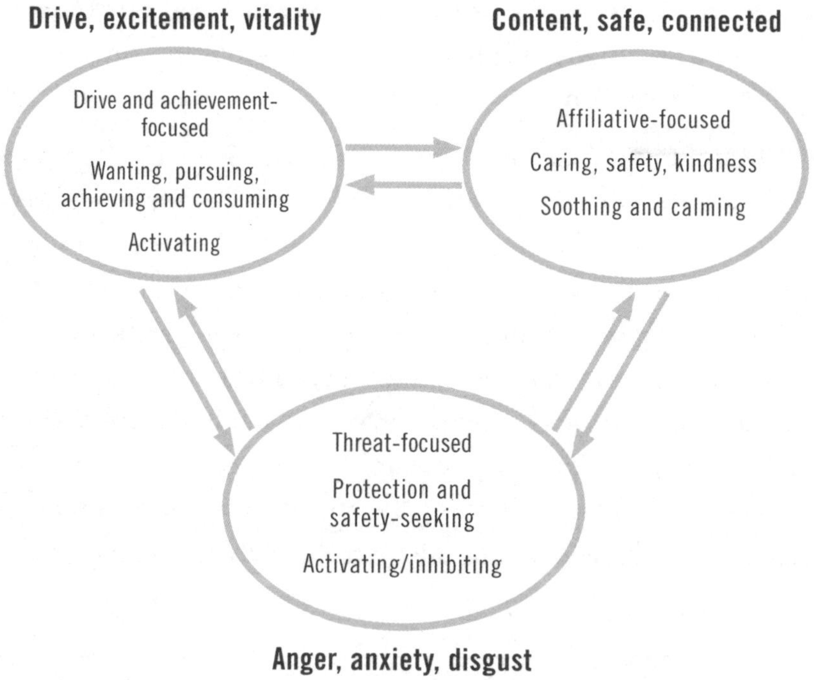

Drive, excitement, vitality   **Content, safe, connected**

Drive and achievement-focused
Wanting, pursuing, achieving and consuming
Activating

Affiliative-focused
Caring, safety, kindness
Soothing and calming

Threat-focused
Protection and safety-seeking
Activating/inhibiting

Anger, anxiety, disgust

Adapted from Gilbert, *The Compassionate Mind* (2009), reprinted with permission from Constable & Robinson Ltd.

The three interacting emotion systems above have much to tell us about compassion, and about training our minds in compassion. We'll return to this in later chapters. For now, let's explore each system in a little more detail.

The threat and self-protection system

The function of this system (known as the threat system for short) is to alert and direct attention to things that are threatening in the world, and motivate us to engage in a response that will protect us and get us to safety. The threat system has a variety of responses it can use to deal with a threat. Upon recognising a threat, this system is linked to a variety of physiological changes in our brain and body that prepare us to take action. It is linked to aspects of our stress response, such as the sympathetic nervous system and the Hypothalamic-Pituitary-Adrenal (HPA) axis that often trigger an energised, activated response. It has a variety of threat emotions associated with it – for example, anger, anxiety and disgust – that urge the body into different patterns of action and response to the threat, often referred to as 'fight or flight'. In terms of behaviour, the threat system urges us to engage in a variety of responses, including aggression, avoidance, submission and so forth. However, at times our threat system will trigger an inhibited or deactivated response. You might have seen a version of this in animals – for example, the mouse that 'plays dead' when in the mouth of a cat but then runs away when it gets the opportunity. This is often referred to as a 'freeze' response.

Threat emotions

Although the threat system is associated with emotions (e.g. anger, anxiety and disgust) that often feel unpleasant, distressing or painful, this doesn't mean the system is 'bad'. It's useful to remember that this system evolved to protect us, and that the emotions linked to it share important functions that support this aim. This is why we refer to them as the *threat emotions*. Take anxiety as an example; this emotion functions to alert us to danger, often motivating us to flee or move away from the threat, or 'freeze' so as not to take us closer to the danger. Think of the feeling you get when walking home in the dark late at night, and you hear footsteps behind you. In comparison, disgust functions to signal us to a threat that might be noxious, toxic or a contaminant, motivating us to move away from it, or clean ourselves. If we eat something that is rotten, disgust may show in expelling this from our bodies (e.g. through spitting it out or even vomiting). Another example of disgust might be the response we have at smelling meat or eggs that have gone off, or when we see certain animals (e.g. cockroaches) or substances (e.g. faeces or vomit) that could be harmful to us. Finally, anger also has a protective function; it often arises when we've experienced a blocked goal or a sense that we've been treated unfairly. Think about patiently waiting for a car parking space, and when it becomes free, another driver sneaking in before you get there. Rather than move away from the situation, you might feel energised to engage with the other driver, by arguing or behaving in a non-verbally aggressive way (e.g. raised voice tone, tense body posture).

Physical and social triggers

What you might have picked up here is that whilst our threat systems function (as they do with other animals) to detect and respond to potential physical threats to our body and life, as a highly social species whose survival and wellbeing is linked to other humans, many of our threats are social in nature. So we know that experiences of rejection, exclusion, criticism and isolation (amongst others) can trigger our threat system, just as they do for other social animals. We will return to this idea later when we think about how our threat systems have been shaped.

Better safe than sorry

Our threat systems are very quick to respond, and will do so outside of conscious (new brain) processing/awareness. Think about your response when, out of the corner of your eye, you see a small dark shape. You might have a quick, automatic flush of fear and tension, maybe even jumping away from it. The fact that it was just a piece of fluff (rather than a spider!) doesn't matter – your mind is programmed respond to the potential of danger first, rather than not responding, taking time to check out what the object is, then making a decision to react. As the saying goes: 'You can have lunch many, many times, but you can only be lunch once'! So our brains and bodies have evolved to take a *better safe than sorry* approach to potential threats in the world. This approach seeks to keep us safe by making quick, 'rough and ready' judgements and responses – even if this means that at times we overestimate the threat.

Under threat conditions, our attention and awareness is directed and 'biased' in a variety of ways. In fact, there are many studies showing that we automatically and quickly pay attention to threat cues over positive cues. For example, in a computer experiment which tracks the movement of eyes, when participants are presented with ninety-nine smiling faces on a screen and one frowning face, they are quicker to spot the scowling face than when presented with one smiling face amongst ninety-nine frowning faces. It might be helpful to consider a more day-to-day example of how this system affects your attention: imagine that you go shopping for a birthday present for a friend or family member. In the first nine shops you go to, the shop assistant is very warm, friendly and helpful. They show you where to find what you are looking for and treat you in a kind way throughout. However, in the tenth and final shop you visit, the shop assistant is very rude to you; they ignore your requests for assistance, talk down to you, and generally appear disrespectful and uninterested in you, or in helping you. When you go home at the end of your shopping day, which of these experiences do you think you will talk about? It is highly likely that though 90 per cent of your experiences were positive, you'd naturally pay attention to, and even ruminate about, the threat-based experiences in the last shop.

We're not suggesting this is a bad thing. Rather, from an evolutionary point of view, it is important that we (like other animals) have ways to pay attention to and prioritise threats in our world. As we discussed above, our brains and bodies have evolved to take a *better safe than sorry* approach to potential threats in the world, and therefore we prioritise these at the expense of positive experiences. This better-safe-than-sorry approach also influences our new brain competencies. So, when our threat systems are triggered, we are more likely to engage in worry, rumination and have our imagination conjure up negative outcomes or interpretations (e.g. worst-case scenarios) than we would experience if our threat systems weren't activated. In understanding how our minds can get caught up in threat-perspectives, it's also important to mention that our brains are very 'plastic', and are shaped by the experiences we have in life. If we experience certain threat-based environments (e.g. bullying, criticism, rejection) that lead to common patterns or loops in the mind (see also Chapter 1), this can lead to ongoing difficulties. Scientists are finding evidence that, like a muscle, the connections between neurons in our brain can become strengthened with frequent use, so under ongoing threat-directed 'loops in the mind', these patterns can become very easily activated. In these scenarios the threat system may now be fuelled 'internally' through these loops, creating an ongoing source of distress and suffering that is separate (although related) to threats we experience in the external world (e.g. people harming, criticising or rejecting us).

It also turns out that if we have a very active threat system, it can be very difficult for us to think about ourselves, other people, and our lives in a balanced and helpful way. We will return to this later in the chapter. Let's consider an example to help us think about what we've learnt about the threat system.

Example: Jenny was in her first term at university. She had found moving away from home very difficult, and was feeling very homesick. In particular, she was struggling to make friends and feel confident. Whether in her lectures, or with her flatmates, she was fearful that other people found her boring and unattractive, and that they didn't want to be friends with her. She often noticed small signs suggesting this, such as someone making a subtle facial expression (e.g. rolling their eyes) or changing the topic of a conversation when she walked in the room.

Jenny described feeling anxious almost all the time around other people, and although she wanted to make friends, she found it difficult to be around people. She would often think of excuses to avoid going out to the pub or to other social events. When she was on her own, she felt less anxious, but still tense, and found herself either worrying about what she would say to people the next time she saw them, or ruminating over recent social interactions where she felt she had made a fool of herself.

So as we can see from Jenny's example, much of her experience of being at university is associated with threat system activation. Key in understanding the influence our threat systems have is to consider how they organise our minds in particular ways. Figure 3.2 opposite highlights this, and you might have noticed from Jenny's example how many different aspects of her mind were directed by her threat system activation. For example, her thinking was skewed to 'worse-case scenarios', and caught in a pattern of worry and rumination. Her behaviour was to stay away from and avoid others where possible, but when with people, her attention was often narrowly focused on small signs that they might not like her or that she had done something wrong (rather than, for example, on times when people had smiled at her or laughed at a joke she had made).

Figure 3.2: Threat system 'organises the mind'

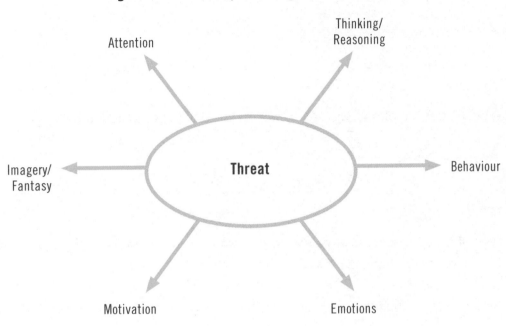

Self-reflection exercise: Given our discussion of the threat system, take some time to think about how this system works for you. The following questions may help you with this.

How often is your threat system triggered?

_____

_____

What things (situations, experiences, thoughts or memories) tend to trigger it?

_____

_____

When activated, how strong (1 being weak, 10 being strong) do you experience this system?

_____

_____

What type of threat emotions (e.g. anger, anxiety) tend to get triggered in these situations?

_____

_____

What type of threat-defence behaviours do you want to engage in when this system is triggered (e.g. aggression, flight, avoidance, submissiveness, etc.)?

_____

_____

What happens to your new brain competencies (e.g. thinking, worrying, ruminating, imagining) when this system is triggered? What type of thoughts do you have?

_____

_____

The drive–excitement system

Although managing threats in the world is a central concern for all animals, there is of course more to life than this alone. In fact, alongside dealing with threats, animals also have to be motivated to pursue resources that would be beneficial to their survival and ultimately, opportunities for reproduction. The emotions and feelings of the drive system – for example, excitement, joy, and anticipation – function to help and energise us to pay attention to, move towards and pursue resources (e.g. food, social status/standing, sexual opportunities) that may be advantageous to us, our offspring, or our group. When these are achieved, this system can leave us with positive emotions and feelings which act as reinforcers, making it more likely that we engage in similar behaviours in the future. In our brains and bodies this system is associated with chemicals that are linked to motivation, activation, reward seeking and pleasure. Like with our threat system, when stimulated, our drive system influences multiple aspects of our minds (see Figure 3.3 below). Let's explore this with the example of Mason.

Example: Mason is a consultant for a large and prestigious management consultancy firm. He worked hard throughout the past year to meet all his targets, and to earn the firm money. His ultimate goal was to earn enough money so that he could buy an engagement ring for his girlfriend. He described feeling very driven and motivated by these goals, and he often spent time thinking about, planning and imagining how to accomplish this.

At his annual review, Mason's manager gave him a lot of positive feedback. She informed Mason that he had been put forward for a promotion (and pay rise), and that he was one of the nominees for the company's annual awards for 'most impressive employee'. After the meeting Mason described feeling 'on top of the world' – full of happiness, excitement and joy. He celebrated the good news with his girlfriend and family in the coming days, appreciating the feedback and reward for his hard work.

Figure 3.3: Drive system 'organises the mind'

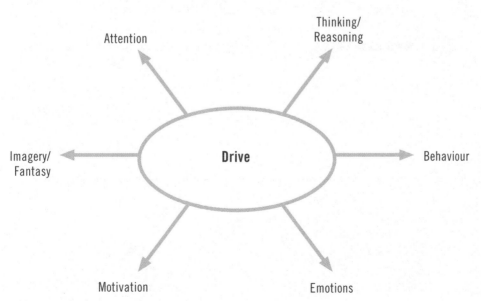

So we can see from Mason's story that he was very drive focused. He had identified goals and 'resources' that were important to him (higher status in the company and more money, to help buy an engagement ring), and his attention, thinking, planning, imagination and crucially, his behaviour, were aligned to enable him to achieve this. Upon achieving this goal Mason experienced excitement, and pleasure for his success.

Self-reflection exercise: Given our discussion of the drive system and Mason's example, take some time to think about how this system works for you. The following questions may help you with this (these can also be found on page 36):

How often is your drive system triggered?

_____

_____

What things (situations, experiences, thoughts or memories) tend to trigger it?

_____

_____

When activated, how strong (1 being weak, 10 being strong) do you experience this system?

_____

_____

What drive emotions (e.g. excitement, joy, happiness) do you experience in these situations?

_____

_____

What type of behaviours do you want to engage in when this system is triggered (e.g. pursuing, getting, celebrating, etc.)?

_____

_____

What happens to your new brain competencies (e.g. thinking, ruminating, imagining and fantasising) when this system is triggered? What type of thoughts do you have?

_____

_____

The soothing–affiliative system

Whilst our threat and drive emotions are essential for our survival and reproduction, if we – as with other animals – were constantly on the move, pursuing, fighting or running away from something, we would soon exhaust ourselves. So it is important that we are able to slow down, rest and recuperate. Returning to our friend the lion from Chapter 1 (page 12), you might have seen on TV that if lions catch a zebra and eat it, they will soon settle down, laze around and sleep. The ability to 'rest and digest' (as this is sometimes referred to) can help to balance the otherwise dominant role that the threat and drive systems would play in our lives. However, this 'soothing system' is not just the product of the absence of threat and drive. It is linked to certain brain and bodily processes (for example, neurohormones such as the opiates and endorphins) that give rise to the pleasant effects of this state – contentment, calmness and peacefulness. The soothing system is therefore linked to a quite different set of positive emotions than those linked to the more activating drive system we discussed earlier.

As we will explore in Chapters 9 and 10, part of Compassionate Mind Training (CMT) involves helping people to create the brain and body (physiological) states involved in safety, calming and contentment. Apart from these being pleasant states to experience in and of themselves, they also allow for an openness and balance in our new brain, facilitating an open, clear and flexible way of thinking. The soothing system is also related to the parasympathetic nervous system, which plays an important role (amongst many others) in regulating and calming our threat systems. As we will see later in the book, this is important as the capacity to slow down and ground oneself may also help us when we need to engage in action (for example, the high-board diver who stills him or herself and takes a number of slower breaths before taking the difficult dive).

The link between the soothing system and care

What is also important for our purposes in Compassionate Mind Training – and in helping you to become more compassionate with yourself – is to understand how evolution has also shaped the soothing system to be highly sensitive to signals of kindness, care and affection from others. As mammals came into the world around 200 million years ago, the soothing system adapted to become tied in to how caring, affection, love and attachment exerted their effects. It's likely that adaptations to the parasympathetic nervous system, along with changes to certain hormones (that ultimately gave rise to two important ones for attachment – vasopressin and oxytocin) meant that the receipt and giving of care now gave a social and relational basis for the soothing system. As we will see later in this chapter, emerging evidence suggests that receiving care, affection and support not only stimulates the soothing system, but also plays a role in down-regulating the threat system. Let's explore this with the example of Lois.

Example: Lois worked hard throughout the week as a teacher, and often found herself in her threat or drive system depending on the class she was giving. Outside of work, she had a number of hobbies – exercising, reading, going to the cinema, and enjoyed socialising with friends. She also made sure she created space and time to slow down, and she often did this through listening to classical music, and regularly practising mindfulness. Lois was also able to turn to others for support and reassurance; recently, she talked to her partner about her difficulties and distress (threat emotions) about a student she was finding difficult to manage in one of her classes. His care, kindness and affection allowed her to settle, calm and feel safe and more at ease. Apart from turning to other people for support and reassurance, Lois was also able to do this internally; she felt able to generate soothing, reassuring and caring inner talk, and this helped her to feel more grounded and able to consider how best to manage this difficult situation at school.

So as we can see from the Lois's example, she was able to access the soothing system in a variety of ways. Not only did she enjoy engaging in relaxing and soothing activities, but crucially, she felt able to turn to others as a source of safety and reassurance. She was also able to turn to herself and tap into a similar sense of internal safety and soothing to manage her distress. As with the threat and drive systems above, when triggered, our soothing system also directs and organises different aspects of our minds, as depicted in Figure 3.4 below.

Figure 3.4: Soothing system 'organises the mind'

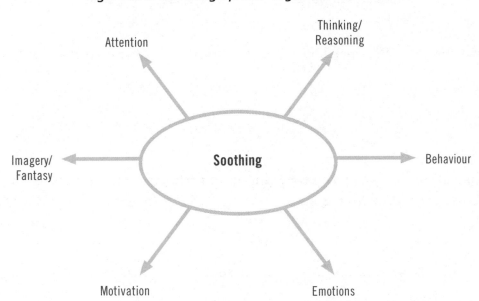

Self-reflection exercise: Given our discussion of the soothing system, take some time to think about how this system works for you. The follow questions may help you with this:

How often is your soothing system triggered?

_____

_____

What things (situations, experiences, thoughts or memories) tend to trigger it?

_____

_____

When activated, how strong (1 being weak, 10 being strong) do you experience this system?

_____

_____

What emotions (e.g. calm, contentment) do you experience in these situations?

_____

_____

What type of behaviours do you want to engage in when this system is triggered (e.g. relaxation, care-giving, care-receiving, etc.)?

_____

_____

What happens to your new brain competencies (e.g. thinking, planning, imagination) when this system is triggered? What type of thoughts do you have?

_____

_____

How are your systems balanced?

It can be helpful at this stage to take some time to think about all three systems together. Take a look at Worksheet 3.1 on page 36, and consider what you've written down for each system. It can also be helpful to answer the following questions.

Is one system triggered more frequently or powerfully than others?

_____

_____

Are any of the systems not experienced very often? Does it feel hard to experience any of these systems?

_____

_____

Exercise: sometimes people find it helpful to consider how each system is balanced in comparison to the others. To do this, take a blank piece of paper and draw out the three circles, using the same structure as in Figure 3.1, page 22 (with threat system at the bottom, drive system top left, and soothing system top right). Draw the size of each circle to reflect how much of this system you experience in your life (so, for example, draw a larger circle for the system that is most dominant in your life, and draw a smaller circle if a system has less of a role or presence). If you find it more helpful, consider the size of each system for particular areas of your life (e.g. a relationship, your job).

After completing this, what are your reflections? Did you learn anything about yourself, or how your systems work? Everyone who completes this exercise will have different experiences, but often a bit of a pattern arises. For example, for many people the threat system seems to be overly active, powerful and long-lasting, whereas the soothing, and sometimes the drive system, are often under-stimulated, or blocked in some way.

Worksheet 3.1 – How your three systems function

	Threat System	Drive System	Soothing System
How often is this system triggered?			
What tends to trigger it?			
How long does it stay activated for once triggered?			
How powerfully do you experience this system when triggered? (1 is weakly, and 10 powerfully)			
What type of thoughts do you have when in this system?			
What do you want to do when this system is triggered?			

What shapes how our three systems function?

Whilst we all share the basic evolved, biological basis of the three emotion systems, we all have slightly different versions of how they function in our lives. There are many reasons for these differences. For example, some of us may inherit genes that might make us more prone to respond to things in an anxious way (threat system), or in reward-seeking or addictive behaviours (drive system). We don't mean to imply that having these innate 'sensitivities' *will* make us respond in a particular way, but that we might be more likely or inclined to do so.

Moreover, these emotion systems are also *learning systems*. This means that they are highly sensitive to the experiences we have in life, so the way they function is dependent on the types of experiences we've had. Let's explore a few ideas around this below.

What experiences in life influence the threat system?

As we explored above, the threat system evolved to help animals pay attention to the presence of threats in the world, and direct appropriate responses accordingly (e.g. fight, flight, freeze or submit) that facilitate safety. Whilst we all have threat systems, the *type* of threat systems we develop depend greatly on the type of experiences we have in life. Here are some examples:

Imagine growing up in a part of the world which was ravaged by civil war – maybe you had experienced bombs exploding close by, or seeing people being shot or even killed, or a general sense that at any moment something bad could happen. You can probably imagine here that your threat system would be learning that the world is a dangerous place, and that you need to be alert and vigilant, in order to respond quickly, if needed.

Imagine that as a child your family have a wonderful dog that you love very much. One day after hurting his paw, your dog bites you painfully on the hand, leaving a nasty bite mark. In this case it is likely that your threat system will learn that dogs are no longer safe, to the extent that next time (and many times after this) you see your dog, or any other dog, you might experience intense feelings of anxiety and the desire to move away from, or even avoid them. In psychological terms, we would refer to this type of learning as 'conditioning'.

Imagine that as a teenager you experience a lot of criticism, shame and hostility from your parents; or that at school, you are bullied quite badly, with people in your year group calling you names, spreading rumours about you and excluding you from a variety of things. These experiences may shape your threat system, alerting you to how people can be threatening, or physically and emotionally hurtful. You may become more anxious and alert to the potential of social or emotional harm to yourself, and worry about how people may treat you in the future. You may even start to feel that this is happening for a reason – that there must be something wrong with you, leading you to blame and criticise yourself. Or, you may become angry and aggressive as a way to protect yourself, as a way of 'getting in there first, before they get you', or blame others for your own difficulties.

Self-reflection exercise: What experiences have affected my threat system?

_____

_____

_____

_____

_____

_____

What experiences in life influence the drive system?

As we outlined previously, the drive system helps us to pay attention to, and energises us towards, things that might be useful or advantageous in some way. Although we all have this system, the way that it works in our lives is highly dependent upon the experiences we've had. Again, it might be helpful here to consider some examples.

Imagine that you are raised by a wealthy family, in an affluent part of a city. Your immediate and extended family are very successful and encouraging people (a high court judge, a professor at a prestigious university, a well-regarded politician), and you attend a private school with lots of children from a similar background. Or imagine that you are raised in a working-class family, with parents who have had to work two jobs each to find a way to pay the bills; that both your parents want you to have a different life to them. They encourage you to study and work hard, and aim 'high' in order to achieve and be successful professionally and financially.

Here's another example. Imagine that your favourite thing in the world is football. As a child you watch every game on TV, and then as a teenager, you begin to realise that you're also a very talented player. You are signed up to the best local team, and your coach tells you that you have a chance to play professionally if you train and practise hard enough. Over the years, you are encouraged and supported by your family, friends and coach to work hard, develop your skills as well as enjoy playing. You play in a very competitive team, against other skilful players, and every time your team wins, or you play well and score, your parents celebrate and praise you for how well you did.

It's likely that in all of these three scenarios – and other similar ones in which striving, achieving and 'having' is valued – your *drive system* will 'hear' these messages, and that as you get older, you will be motivated to (and enjoy) achieving things, whatever they may be.

Self-reflection exercise: What experiences have shaped my drive system?

_____

_____

_____

_____

_____

_____

It's also worth pointing out here about *threat-based drive*. This involves a drive-based focus but underpinned by the threat system. For example, imagine growing up in a house in which achievements and success were highly valued, but at the same time non-achievement brought disappointment, criticism or even anger from your parents, family or school teachers. Imagine how this might leave you feeling. Here, it is possible that striving and trying to achieve comes with a background flavour of stress or anxiety. Interestingly, research conducted by one of us (Chris Irons) with Paul Gilbert and other colleagues found that striving to achieve to avoid feelings of inferiority was associated with higher levels of depression, anxiety and stress symptoms.

Self-reflection exercise: have you had any experiences of threat-based drive? If so, what experiences have you had that might have shaped this system?

_____

_____

_____

_____

_____

What experiences in life influence the soothing-affiliative system?

Humans, like other mammals, provide care to their young in a variety of forms, including protection, feeding, shelter, affection, distress reduction, and so forth. Evidence now suggests that the quality of this care – both in our early years and throughout our lives – influences the functioning of the soothing-affiliative system. So, if you're lucky enough to have parents who are very attentive, affectionate, consistent and nurturing, it's likely that these experiences build capacity in the soothing system, which in turn gives rise to the potential for a number of other important things. First, we associate other people with a sense of safety – that they will be there for us when needed, that they can soothe our distress and pain, that they can help us to contain and make sense of our feelings. Second, these experiences lay down emotional memories that, over time, make us able to soothe and calm our own distress. Third, these experiences may provide groundedness, safeness and confidence to move into the world and engage in exploration – to do things we value and enjoy, or even facing challenges from which we might benefit. In other words, this system can help us access our drive system.

Now, imagine for a moment that you are raised in a family that for whatever reason is not able to treat you with care, affection and support. Imagine if, when you are distressed, others don't respond in a helpful way, but instead with hostility and anger, or hardly respond at all. How might this affect you? Our clinical experience, along with the research literature, suggests that the absence of these experiences can leave people having to manage the world and their emotions through different routes, often linked to the strategies of the threat or drive systems. Here are a couple of examples to consider.

Example: Deborah is the youngest of three sisters, and was brought up by her mother. Sadly, her father died in a car crash before she was born. Whilst her mother could be very loving at times, she was often very stressed trying to look after three children whilst also working full-time in a demanding job to pay the bills. Although Deborah didn't realise it at the time, she found out later that her mother suffered from regular and quite severe bouts of depression. Although never nasty or threatening to her, Deborah could not remember her mother showing her much warmth, affection or love.

Example: Richard was an only child, and grew up with his mother and father. He recalled that his father was often away for long periods of time for work, whilst his mother had a part-time job at the local school. Richard had very clear memories of his mother caring for him – being tactile, affectionate and very loving. However, he also recalled periods of time when she would react in unpredictable ways – for example, with coldness rather than warmth and affection, or promises to do things with him that she was unable to keep. Growing up, Richard found it hard to rely on other people, with a sense they might let him down, or suddenly turn away from him, or even against him.

In both of these examples it is likely that Deborah and Richard's soothing systems have been adversely affected by their experiences. In other words, the soothing systems may not have had the inputs/learning to help them fully develop with an underlying sense of instability and difficulty trusting feelings of connection and safety.

Self-reflection: What experiences have shaped my soothing system?

_____

_____

_____

_____

_____

Summary: how our three systems have been shaped

Sometimes when we spend time reflecting on how our three systems have been shaped it can be quite illuminating – almost like things 'click', and we understand why our emotions are like they are. For some people, this exercise can make them sad about things that have happened in life, maybe even the loss of certain experiences or relationships. Whilst this might be painful, it may help us to recognise that parts of our lives have been difficult and not how we would have liked them to be. This may, in turn, be an important step towards understanding why practising and developing compassion for ourselves may be helpful.

What can CMT do to help?

Hopefully the above description of the three-system model makes sense, and you can see how they might apply in your life. For many people, it is quite clear to see that they are out of balance, often with over-activation of the threat system, problems with the drive system (either it becoming too strong or blocked in some way), and commonly, an underactive or blocked soothing-affiliative system.

In Compassionate Mind Training (CMT) we are interested in how we can bring *balance* to these different systems. The aim is not to get rid of any of them, but rather to see if we can:

- Understand why the systems work in the way they do

- Understand how they impact on each other

- Consider ways to reduce those that may be over-active and causing us difficulties (e.g. the threat system)

- Build the soothing-affiliative system

- Develop compassion as a way of bringing the systems into greater balance.

There are a variety of specific things that we can do to help with this, and we will explore these throughout the rest of the book.

Why focus on developing the soothing-affiliative system?

There is increasing evidence that the soothing-affiliative system, including the experiences that stimulate it (e.g. giving and receiving of affection, kindness and care), along with the feelings it stimulates (e.g. warmth, calmness, contentment), may naturally help to regulate or balance the activity of the threat system. For example, we now know that oxytocin, the hormone we mentioned earlier, seems to have a natural soothing impact on the stress hormones and areas of the brain associated with the threat system.

There are some interesting studies showing the relationship between the two. For example, in one study, researchers asked married women to come to the lab to have their brains scanned. At various times during the scan, the women were given mild electric shocks. As you can imagine, upon receiving the electric shocks, participants responded with fear. On the brain scan, areas of the brain associated with threat were activated/lit up. In another part of the experiment, the women's husbands were present, holding their hands while the electric shocks were given. This time, the researchers noticed that the threat response in the brain was reduced. Interestingly, the higher the women rated the quality of their relationship, the greater the reduction in threat activation in their brain scans.

It's important here to highlight that the soothing-affiliative system does not only calm or reduce the power of the threat system, or bring a sense of contentment. Whilst these are important functions of the system, it is what this system facilitates that's important to us. Consider the following example: imagine that whilst having a shower, you've notice a lump on your body that wasn't there the last time you checked, and that you start worrying that you might have cancer. Each time you think about this lump – and what it might be – you feel very anxious and worried that you might die (your threat system is activated). You're so worried that you try to avoid thinking about the lump, or doing anything about it. In fact, you have been procrastinating about booking an appointment to see the doctor, even though you know this would be the wisest thing to do. Now, imagine that you've got someone in your life who cares for you deeply; someone who is reliable, strong and warm. Imagine that this person has found out about the lump, and is there to support and help you with your fear. How do you think this will affect what you do? For many of us, having supportive people in our lives helps to reduce our sense of threat, and encourages us to take difficult steps forward. So, the soothing-affiliative system has an important role to play in helping us manage our threat system, by allowing us to feel calm, content and at ease, as well as empowering us to take action in difficult circumstances.

It is sometimes the case that we do not have such soothing, supportive people in our lives to help us in these situations. Moreover, some of us struggle to engage this system for ourselves. What we mean by this is that, through no fault of our own, we can have great difficulty activating this system to self-soothe and help ourselves through difficult times, because we have not had the life experiences that give rise to the soothing-affiliative system. This difficulty is a key concern for Compassionate Mind Training (CMT), and throughout this book we will spend time helping you to develop the capacity to 'self-soothe'.

Chapter summary

In this chapter we learned about our emotions, and what function they have evolved to play in our lives.

What we have learnt together	My personal reflections on the chapter
1. We have three basic emotion systems: threat, drive and soothing. 2. Each of these systems – and the emotions that go with them – has different functions. 3. The threat emotions function to alert us to potential danger, or blocks to our goals, and urge us to take appropriate responses. 4. The drive emotions function to make us pay attention to opportunities that might be beneficial to us, and motivate us to pursue and acquire resources. 5. The soothing system helps us to experience periods of calmness, contentment and safety, and is particularly sensitive to the care and affiliation of others. 6. Our emotion systems are shaped by our experiences. They can often get out of balance, which can skew our emotions, thoughts, attention, behaviour, etc. in a particular way (often in a threat- or drive-based way). 7. CMT can help us to bring greater balance to our emotion systems, through developing the soothing-affiliative system, in particular.	

4 Understanding how and why our difficulties arise

'It is wisdom to know others; it is enlightenment to know one's self.'

– Lao-Tzu

So far we've explored ideas about how we can encounter difficulties in life – for example, through having tricky brains that get easily caught up in loops, or having our emotion systems out of balance. We've also considered how we have all been shaped by the experiences we've had in life, and how these may have also led to difficulties for some of us. In this chapter, we're going to bring some of these ideas together and work on helping you to understand your difficulties and the things you struggle with day-to-day.

In this chapter, we will:

- Look at the reasons why you might be struggling at the moment

- Consider how these difficulties might be maintained in a number of understandable ways

- Consider how we can start to bring compassion to our difficulties.

Why is understanding our difficulties important?

On one level, it is probably quite obvious why gaining an understanding of our difficulties might be important. Just as it would be important for your GP to try and understand the nature and causes of your stomach pain to be able to provide the right treatment, the more we understand the nature of our psychological difficulties, how our minds work and how these have been shaped by our environment, the more likely we are to find effective ways of addressing them. In psychological therapy, this process is often called a *formulation*. A formulation is a way of using information about a person – for example, the nature of their difficulties and history – and forming an understanding based on psychological theory, to offer hypotheses about the cause and maintenance of their difficulties.

As well as having a helpful formulation, in Compassionate Mind Training (CMT) we are particularly interested in how we can bring a compassionate understanding to the development and maintenance of our difficulties, and how compassion may help us to make changes, and move forward.

There are three main types of formulation in CMT:

- Understanding the loops in our mind (old brain-new brain)

- Understanding how our three emotion systems are balanced (three-system model)

- Understanding how the threat-focused brain can 'run the show' and keep us locked in patterns developed through experiences in the past.

We have already explored many aspects of the first two of these in Chapters 1 and 3, and it might be helpful just to spend a moment familiarising yourself with these again before continuing.

In this chapter we are going to explore the third type of formulation. If it helps, you might choose to ask a friend or family member who knows you well (and with whom you feel safe) to help you to complete it. Because this chapter focuses on our life history and how this has influenced us, it can sometimes be quite an emotional process. It can therefore be helpful to take this chapter in stages – working on a bit, taking a break or a small breather, and returning to it when you feel ready. It can also be helpful to chat to someone you feel safe with if it does evoke any strong feelings in you. Remember, you can always return to this chapter later if you find that more helpful, and sometimes people find it easier to engage with once they've developed more compassionate mind skills that we look at in Sections III and IV.

Many people find working on their own formulation very helpful, although sometimes challenging. We know this partly because of what our patients have told us over the many years of practising CMT. But we also know because we have used these formulations to understand our own difficulties as well, and therefore know a bit about what the process is like. We will help you to develop your formulation below, in a step-by-step way. To assist with this, we've also outlined the formulation of Emma – someone who came for therapy wanting to find a way to change her life and not feel so depressed.

Example: Emma came to therapy as she had been feeling depressed and anxious for the past three months, after finding out that her partner had been unfaithful to her. She described feeling overwhelmed by this, and that she blamed herself for him cheating, as 'there must have been something wrong with me for why he did it'. She also described feeling very lonely, with a sense that other people couldn't be trusted, particularly as people had hurt or rejected her in the past.

Emma was born and raised in Edinburgh. She recalled how her parents often argued a lot, and that her Dad was often angry and critical towards her. Whilst her mother was kinder, she was often emotionally detached, and Emma wondered whether she had also suffered from depression. At school, Emma had some friends, but was also bullied, and whilst she achieved good exam results, compared herself negatively to her sister, who achieved straight A grades. Emma went to university, but didn't enjoy the subject she took (Business Studies) or being away from home. Since graduating, she has been working at a large company as a business consultant, but really dislikes her job, and would like to leave.

During her third session in therapy, Emma was helped to use some of the above information (along with other information she gave about her current and early life) to develop a formulation of how her life experiences had influenced her current difficulties now. You can see a copy of Emma's formulation in Worksheet 4.1 (page 49). We will explore specific aspects of Emma's formulation in a step-by-step way, below.

There are five main steps in helping to understand our difficulties. We will explore each of these in turn, giving you an opportunity to think about how each step relates to your own experiences. We will also use Emma as an example, so that we can see how this worked for her.

Step 1: Historical influences

When stressful, painful or frightening things happen to us – especially as children – our brain automatically shifts to a threat and protection mode. We may become anxious, wary of others and learn to keep our distance/try to 'keep our head down', or we could become quite angry, prone to aggression and even episodes of violence. Later, these tendencies can become easily triggered and as a consequence, cause problems for ourselves and others.

So the first step of the formulation process (Worksheet 4.1) involves reflecting on the key negative/difficult experiences in your life that have influenced us (this links to what we discussed in Chapter 2, see pages 16–20), and the development of our threat system. These may be things that happened early in our lives – like the death of a close family member, or not experiencing warmth or affection from our parents, or experiencing abuse from someone who cared for us. It could be things that happened during adolescence – for example, being bullied at school, struggling to fit in with our peer group, or experiencing a failure or setback in some way (e.g. at a sports trial or exams). It may be that these experiences occurred later in life; for example, finding out that our partner was unfaithful, or failing an important exam.

When filling out Worksheet 4.1, often we are focusing on some of the difficult things that have happened to us, and those in particular that have stimulated our threat system. Sometimes it can be helpful to consider whether there were any difficult experiences in any of the following areas:

Relationships: For example, with mum, dad, siblings, extended family, friends and romantic/sexual partners. These might include experiencing criticism, blame, anger or aggression, rejection or a sense of intrusion. They may also include an experience that others were absent or unavailable, or that they lacked affection, care or kindness towards you.

School: Including experiences of struggling academically/not achieving what self or others expected; being bullied or not fitting in.

Employment: Including feeling that we haven't achieved enough at work, of being bullied by our boss or colleagues, of losing our job or being passed over for promotion.

So, when you feel ready, spend a little time writing down some of your key experiences in life in the table below. Don't feel you have to write things out in full sentences. For example, if you write down 'Dad – uncaring' or 'Friends – unpredictable' it's likely that you'll remember exactly what this means without having to write it out in full. As a guide, we've given examples of Emma's early life experiences. Your experiences may be similar to hers, or very different.

Worksheet 4.1: My background/experiences

Emma's background/experiences	My background/experiences
Identified a number of key experiences in life that she felt might have affected or influenced her.	Think about the experiences that you've had in life that may have impacted or affected you. Make notes about the following areas:
Early family relationships	*Early family relationships*
• Parents argued a lot, Dad was often physically violent and critical • Parents divorced when I was eight years old – felt it was my fault they separated • Mum could be caring but often was detached and emotionally cold. Felt as if her job was more important than me • Parents favoured my sister because she was smarter than me.	
School/academic experiences	*School/academic experiences*
• Enjoyed primary school, but didn't like secondary school – I was bullied about my appearance and being last in my class to get my period • I did OK in my exams but Mum always responded with: 'Almost as good as your sister' • Didn't enjoy university – others more intelligent and popular than me.	
Peer/romantic relationships	*Peer/romantic relationships*
• Fell in love with Steve when – sixteen – first boyfriend – found out he had been cheating on me whole time.	
Career experiences	*Career experiences*
Not enjoying my job – passed over for promotion a number of times.	

Step 2: Considering how your background experiences have affected your threat system

As we explored in Chapters 2 and 3, the experiences we have in life influence and shape us in a variety of ways. In our formulation, Step 2 involves thinking about how the type of experiences you've had (those that you've highlighted in Worksheet 4.1) might have affected you – how they might have led to you developing certain key fears, threats or concerns that you still experience in your life now. In a sense, it is considering how the things that we've been through have influenced, shaped or affected our threat system.

Box 4.1: Some tips to help with common fears and threats

Tips – some common fears and threats

As CMT takes the view that we all have a brain that evolved to be sensitive to certain types of stressors and dangers in the world, it might not come as a surprise to you that there are often some common types of threats and fears that people report. These include:

External Fears

(our concerns about how others may think, feel or treat us)

- Rejection – fearing that others will turn us away, or not accept, our attempts for connection and/or affection and that we will be unwanted

- Abandonment – a fear that others will withdraw their connection and support

- Exclusion – a sense that others will actively keep us disconnected from them or others (e.g. friends, colleagues)

- Distrust – that others cannot be trusted, that they will betray, let us down or be untruthful with us

- Harm – that others may intentionally hurt us (e.g. physical or emotional)

- Criticism or ridicule – that other people will be critical, shaming or look down on us

Internal Fears

(our concerns about things that arise inside of us)

- Identity concerns – for example, feeling that we are unworthy, not good enough or a failure

- Emotions/feelings – for example, concerns that our feelings might overwhelm us, or that if we allow ourselves to experience them, they might never end. We may have a sense that emotions are 'bad', dangerous or a sign of 'weakness'. We may feel this about all emotions and feelings, or about specific ones (e.g. anger, sadness)

- Memories – of bad things that have happened to us in the past that keep intruding into our minds in the present day

- Aloneness or loneliness – a sense of feeling disconnected or separate from others, but with an underlying wish for connection

In CMT, we try and split these fears and threats between those that are *external* to us (that is, threats in the world or other people), and those that are *internal* (that is, they arise inside of us, such as our emotions, or feelings about ourselves). This distinction might seem a little tricky to begin with. We've given a few tips regarding fears and threats in Box 4.1 above and we'll have a look at Emma's key external and internal fears, as well. After that, have a go at completing Worksheet 4.2 overleaf and log your own key threats and fears.

Worksheet 4.2: My key fears and threats

Emma's key fears and threats	My key fears and threats
Given Emma's background, we identified a number of key fears and threats that had left her struggling.	After reading through the example of Emma, have a think about yourself. Given your experiences in life, what are your key external and internal threats?
Emma's external fears/threats (things she feared others might think about her, or do to her) included:	My *external fears/threats* are ...
• Others can't be trusted (this was particularly linked to being cheated on by her first boyfriend)	
• Others will reject me (this was linked to the experience of her dad being absent, and her boyfriend leaving her)	
• Others will look down on me/are critical of me (this was linked to experiencing her mum being critical, and her peers as shaming).	
We were also able to outline a number of key *internal fears* (things that emerged inside her that were uncomfortable or threatening). These included:	My *internal fears/threats* are ...
• I am not good enough (linked to the experience that her sister was favoured and 'smarter')	
• My emotions are overwhelming and too painful (this was related to her parents being emotionally detached, and to mum criticising her when she expressed strong emotions as a child)	
• I am alone and lonely (this was linked to feeling that she had always been separate from others – her mum, sister and friends).	

Step 3: How have you tried to protect yourself from your fears?

So far we have explored how our experiences in life may have played a role in leading to things that we find difficult and threatening now. Step 3 in this process is for us to consider how, given the fears that you have jotted down in Worksheet 4.2, you might have engaged in strategies to cope with these fears – what we refer to as *protective* or *safety strategies*. These protective strategies are things that, over the years, you might have learned to use, or just stumbled upon and then continued to use. It is likely that to some extent, these strategies have helped you in some way to manage, deal with, reduce or minimise the threats that you experience in column 2. In our experience, they are often strategies that if we were to think about someone else who experiences similar types of key threats and concerns as we do, we could see (and maybe even empathise with) why these strategies had developed as an understandable way of dealing with difficulties in life.

To help us think about this, it is helpful for us to return back to Emma again, and see what strategies she identified using to manage her fears and threats. When you've had a look through the strategies she uses, have a think about your own protective strategies and note these down in Worksheet 4.3. It might also be helpful to look at Box 4.2 below for some common examples of protective strategies.

Box 4.2: Some tips to help with common protective and safety strategies

Tips – some common protective and safety strategies

Similarly to the fears and threats, it turns out that there are also some common safety or protective strategies that many of us use. Many of these are linked to how other animals manage threats – for example, through evolved defences of freeze, flight, fight, submission and so forth. Again, we can split these between common strategies used to manage external fears, and those used to manage internal fears:

Protective strategies used to manage external fears

- Avoidance – for example, of getting close to people or anxiety-provoking situations
- Relying on self, rather than on others

- Submissiveness – 'keeping your head down', being passive and not asserting yourself

- Hypervigilance – trying to spot external threats as quickly as possible, so that they can be dealt with

- Seeking reassurance from, or closeness with, others.

Protective strategies to manage internal fears

- Suppression of feelings or emotions (trying not to 'feel' difficult things)

- Striving to succeed to feel like we are worthy (e.g. trying to achieve/be the best)

- Self-criticism – we can beat ourselves up for things we don't like about ourselves (for example, as a way of trying to improve ourselves)

- Try to connect with others/be closer to others, to reduce feelings of aloneness.

Worksheet 4.3: Safety and protective strategies

Emma's safety and protective strategies	My safety and protective strategies
After identifying her key fears and threats, we went on to outline ways that Emma had helped to protect herself from these.	Whilst holding in mind the key external fears and threats you noted down in Worksheet 4.2 (page 52), what are the protective strategies you use to keep yourself safe from your fears?
To protect herself from her *external fears* that others could not be trusted, that others would reject her, and that others would look down on her/be critical, Emma reported: - Keeping my distance from others - Keeping on guard and vigilant of what others might do/think - Trying to please other people so they won't hurt or reject me.	My safety strategies to protect against external fears are:

To protect herself from her *internal fears* of not being good enough, having overwhelming emotions, and feeling alone, Emma identified:

- Trying not to strive or push myself, for fear that I'll fail if I did

- Suppressing and keeping my feelings to myself

- Using food and alcohol as a way to not feel distress.

Now, have a read through what you noted down for internal fears in Worksheet 4.2. Given this, how do you protect yourself from these?

Step 4: Exploring whether there are any unintended consequences of the safety strategies you often use

Step 4 is about trying to acknowledge and explore how, whilst often helpful to a certain extent (or often when used in the short term), our protective strategies can lead to some unintended or unpleasant consequences – a bit like downsides or side effects. One of the key things here is to understand and appreciate that these consequences are *unintended*. What we mean here is that, when we started to use our protective strategies (which for some of us could have been many, many years ago!), it's unlikely that we knew that by doing so, these would lead to difficulties down the line. Rather, we used them because on one level, they helped to reduce the distress related to our external and internal fears. Moreover, it is unlikely that we chose these strategies consciously – we probably didn't say: 'Now that I've turned fifteen, I've decided that I'm going to start suppressing my feelings, as this will help to block out my painful emotions'! The reality is that these protective strategies develop over time and are rarely consciously 'chosen'; rather, we may become conscious of them later on in life, often when they no longer work.

Box 4.3: Some tips to help with common unintended consequences

---

Tips – some common unintended consequences linked to protective strategies

External

- If I try to avoid others (safety strategy), I am left feeling alone and unwanted (unintended consequence)
- If I try to appease other people (safety strategy), this might leave me feeling that my needs are not met.

Internal

- Blaming myself for bad things that happen (safety strategy) might leave me feeling low in self-esteem and mood (unintended consequence)
- Suppressing my feelings (safety strategy) leaves me experiencing those feelings more frequently and powerfully (known as the bounce-back effect, and in this instance, an unintended consequence).

So again, we would like you to have a go at noting any of your own unintended consequences in Worksheet 4.4 below based on the protective strategies that you noted in step 3. Again, it might be helpful to have a look at Emma's unintended consequences, to see the sort of things she noted about her life. It may also be helpful to look at Box 4.3 for some tips on common unintended consequences.

Worksheet 4.4: My unintended consequences

Emma's unintended consequences	My unintended consequences
After identifying her safety strategies, we then went on to help Emma identify whether these strategies had any unintended consequences. Following her strategies of keeping her distance from people, staying on guard and pleasing others so as to manage her external fears, Emma identified the following unintended consequences: • The more I keep my distance from others, the more lonely I feel • The more I stay on guard, the more suspicious I am of other people's intentions • The more I try and please others, the more my own needs don't get met. We also looked at the unintended consequences that followed from the safety strategies that she uses – not pushing herself, suppressing her feelings and self-harm – to manage her internal fears. Emma identified: • The more I don't push myself, the more I feel like a failure • The more I suppress my feelings, the more I get overwhelmed with them • When I self-harm, I get scars and these leave me feeling ashamed.	Having looked through the example of Emma, and going through your safety strategies in Worksheet 4.3 (page 54), consider whether you have experienced any unintended consequences from these. *My unintended consequences from external safety strategies* *My unintended consequences from internal safety strategies*

Step 5: Feedback loops

So, looking at the fourth column of your formulation, it can be useful to reflect on two questions:

- How are you left feeling about yourself – what your 'self-to-self' relationship is – when you read through the unintended consequences in column four?

- What tends to happen to your mood, feelings or symptoms when you read through the unintended consequences?

As you can see from Emma's formulation example in Figure 4.1, the unintended consequences in her life (column 4) left her feeling more critical of herself – she disliked herself and, at times, even described hating the person that she had become. Understandably, the combination of her unintended consequences as well as this critical way of thinking about herself left her feeling low in mood.

To finish the process, we asked Emma to reflect on column 4. When she experienced the type of unintended consequences she did, along with an increase in self-criticism and lower mood, what happened to the key fears and threats she had noted down in column 2? As the 'arrow' indicates, these feelings had the effect of creating a feedback loop back to her key fears and threats, 'heating them up'. Of course, the stronger Emma's fears were in column 2, the more she felt she needed to engage in her protective strategies (column 3), which in turn, made it more likely that she would experience unintended consequences from these. So, in effect, a feedback loop is created that continues to fuel her distress.

Think about this process for yourself. Given your unintended consequences, how do you feel about yourself? Do you have similar self-critical thoughts as Emma did? What happens to your mood if this is the case? And how does the way in which you relate to yourself (column 4), impact upon your fears and threats (column 2)?

Figure 4.1: Emma's Formulation

Key Historical Influences	Key Fears/Threats	Protective/Safety Strategies	Unintended Consequences
• Parents divorced when I was eight years old – before that they argued a lot and Dad was physically violent to Mum	**External**	**External**	**External**
• Mum was caring at times, but her work came before me. Often detached and emotionally cold	Others are untrustworthy	Keep my distance	Lonely
• Dad worked away a lot for business – when around, he was angry and critical	Other people will reject me	Keep on guard – wary of others	Suspicious of others' intentions
• Sister (two years older) – always achieving and popular; felt parents favoured her	Others look down on me	Try to please	Don't get needs met
• Enjoyed primary school, but felt out of depth in secondary school – felt alone much of the time and was bullied for being the last in my year to go through puberty	**Internal**	**Internal**	**Internal**
• Did well in exams, but Mum responded with 'Almost as good as your sister'	Not good enough	Don't push self/strive	Not achieve/feel like a failure
• Fell in love at sixteen with first boyfriend – relationship lasted one year but found out that he had been unfaithful most of the time	Emotions overwhelming (especially sadness and anger)	Keep feelings to self	Get overwhelmed with strong feelings
• Struggled at university – didn't enjoy subject and felt others more intelligent and popular than me	Alone	Overeat and use alcohol	Gain weight – feel ashamed of self and body
• Employed for the past three years in junior role at large company – not enjoying job but feel unable to leave – I'd be seen as a failure			**Self-to-self relating**
			Criticise and hate myself →
			Mood
			Depressed, sad, hate life →

Worksheet 4.5: My Formulation

Key Historical Influences (What key historical experiences have influenced you?)	Key Fears/Threats (Given historical experiences, what key fears have you been left with?)	Protective/Safety Strategies (Given key fears, what safety strategies have you developed to protect yourself?)	Unintended Consequences (Have your safety strategies led to any unintended or unforeseen consequences?)
	External	External	External
	Internal	Internal	Internal
			→ Self-to-self relating → Mood

Bringing it all together

At this stage it might be helpful to bring together all of the five steps we've been working on in this chapter. On page 60 you will see a blank version of the formulation (Worksheet 4.5), and the completed form that Emma did. Just like she did, we would like you to write down the different answers you've noted down during this chapter. Take your time with this, and remember you can use Emma's formulation as a guide for your own (you may have similar or different themes, but hopefully can see how her formulation makes sense). If it helps, speak to someone that you trust – maybe a friend or family member – who might be able to guide you with this process.

Self-reflection exercise: How did you find trying to formulate yourself?

So, how did you find trying to develop a formulation of your own difficulties? What did you learn about your current struggles, and their origins? How did this discovery leave you feeling?

_____

_____

_____

_____

Common difficulties during formulation

As we mentioned at the start of this chapter, it can be difficult to complete our own formulation. There are a number of common reasons for this:

Negative feelings: Sometimes when we think about our difficulties using the focus described above we may feel more anxious or low in mood. Sometimes we can begin to feel sad or upset, recognising that life has been quite hard.

Not being able to write anything down: Sometimes we can feel reluctant to write anything down, almost as if writing it down is some sort of betrayal to other people. For example, Sarah struggled to write anything down in the first column (difficult life experiences) as she felt that doing this would be betraying her parents. This sense of disloyalty made it hard for her to connect emotionally with some of the experiences she had growing up at home. On the other hand, Dan struggled to put anything in column 1 (background experiences), as initially he couldn't think of anything 'bad enough' that had happened to him to cause him problems. He struggled to see that his current problems were 'valid' given his earlier experiences, and felt that people only became depressed if they'd gone through 'really awful things'.

Finding it difficult to know what to write: For some people, it's difficult to know exactly what to put down in the formulation. For example, whilst Ben was able to make some notes about some of his key experiences in life (column 1), he found it difficult to know what key threats this had led him to experience now (column 2). For others, the struggle to work out what to write is linked to wanting to get the 'right' thing down – a type of perfectionism that can block us from connecting with the process of formulation.

Separating external to internal threats: In our experience one of the most common difficulties in doing this type of formulation is in working out which threats (column 2) are external, and which are internal. Of course, this distinction is somewhat arbitrary but can be helpful if we are able to separate them, as the way in which we try to help ourselves with external threats might be quite different to how we deal with internal ones. Try not to worry too much about these distinctions if it feels like they're getting in the way – the key thing is to try and connect with some of the key fears or threats that you're experiencing at the moment.

Bringing compassion to your formulation

If you struggled with any of the above experiences during formulation (or any others for that matter), please try to remember it may be helpful to take a step back, speak to a friend or someone you feel safe with, or do something else that helps when you feel upset (e.g. going for a walk, reading a book), before coming back to it when you feel able to.

If you can, try not to be too hard on yourself with this – it is often the case that when we look more closely at some of the struggles we have, we feel worse. The saying 'out of sight, out of mind' is interesting – maybe when it comes to focusing on our difficulties during formulation the intention is 'in sight, in mind' - but that can trigger our threat system and result in distress. Try and remember that whilst completing your formulation might have been tricky or distressing, you're not the only one. Along with many other people we have completed our own formulations and found some of this difficult as well. It may be helpful to hold onto the reason why we are doing this – our compassionate intention to become more sensitive to our difficulties and distress, and to develop skills that may help alleviate these and move us forward in life.

However, once we have completed our formulations, it can be helpful to try to look at them through a particular perspective. This is where we are going to bring compassion to guide our way of understanding our formulation. Have a look at Figure 4.2 overleaf to get an idea of how Emma started to think about compassion on her formulation. In terms of your compassion training, we are still in the early stages so don't worry if this all feels a little bit too much to take in. Below we're going to help you to start bringing the first steps of compassion to your own formulation.

Maybe you can also try out the following:

Is it possible at all to see why things are like they are for you? Why your key fears developed given your early experiences? Why it makes sense that you tried to manage these fears and threats by developing a variety of safety strategies? And why, although helpful in places, these safety strategies have led to certain unintended consequences?

Self-reflection: _____

_____

_____

_____

Figure 4.2: Bringing Compassion to Emma's Formulation

Key Historical Influences (What key historical experiences have influenced you?)	Key Fears/Threats (Given historical experiences, what key fears have you been left with?)	Protective/Safety Strategies (Given key fears, what safety strategies have you developed to protect yourself?)	Unintended Consequences (Have your safety strategies led to any unintended or unforeseen consequences?)
• Parents divorced when I was eight years old – before that they argued a lot and Dad was physically violent to Mum • Mum was caring at times, but felt her work came before being interested in me. Often detached and emotionally detached and cold • Dad away a lot – was angry and critical when there • Sister (two years older) – always achieving and popular; felt parents favoured her • Enjoyed primary school but felt out of depth in large secondary school – bullied for being the last in my year to go through puberty • Did well in exams, but Mum responded with 'Almost as good as your sister' • Fell in love at sixteen with first boyfriend – relationship lasted one year but found out that he had been unfaithful most of the time • Struggled at university – didn't enjoy subject and felt others more intelligent and popular than me • Employed for the past three years in junior role at large company – not enjoying job but feel unable to leave for fear that would be seen as a failure.	**External** Others are untrustworthy Other people will reject me Others look down on me **Internal** Not good enough Emotions overwhelming (especially sadness and anger) Alone	**External** Keep my distance Keep on guard – vigilant of others Try to please **Internal** Don't push self/strive Keep feelings to self Overeat and use alcohol	**External** Lonely Suspicious of others' intentions Don't get needs met **Internal** Not achieve/feel like a failure Get overwhelmed with strong feelings Gain weight – feel ashamed of self and body **Self-to-self relating** Criticise and hate myself **Mood** Depressed, sad, hate life
• Empathy and understanding that I did not choose these experiences but they had a big impact on the development of a version of me • Not my fault • Validate that these were difficult experiences	• Understandable why these threats/fears developed • Others are likely to have these fears, given same genes/ experiences	• Understandable that developed strategies to deal with fears • These strategies have helped me at times	• Although helpful at times, I can see that safety strategies led to some unintended consequences

Bringing a Compassionate Mind to the Formulation

If you considered that a friend had experienced what you did, what fears might they have developed in life? Could you imagine that they might have similar types of fears – and maybe developed similar types of safety strategies, with similar unintended consequences, as you have? Would you feel critical or blaming of them for any of their struggles? Or are you able to see that there are understandable reasons for why this is like that?

Self-reflection: _____

_____

_____

_____

Some of these points above might be difficult, but they may also help you to understand (and develop greater empathy) for why you're struggling with what you're struggling with. A little like imagining having to run a marathon (26.2 miles) after doing just one practice run (of 1 mile!), it might be that trying to bring compassion to your formulation feels impossible at this stage. Again, try not to worry too much if this is the case – this is just a starting point, and we will return to working on this when you feel like you've had more chance to develop your strength and skills in compassion.

Chapter summary

In this chapter we have looked at what formulation is, reviewed an example of a formulation (Emma's), and given some space for you to think about how you would formulate your own difficulties. We have also looked at how thinking about our own difficulties and trying to understand the context in which they developed, can be challenging. We finished the chapter by exploring how we might hold these difficulties as understandable and try to bring a compassionate approach to our struggles.

What we have learnt together	My personal reflections on the chapter
In this chapter, we have: 1. Explored how we can understand the development and maintenance of our difficulties based on the experiences we've had in life (called a 'formulation'). 2. Provided an opportunity for you to have a go at formulating your own difficulties. 3. Considered how bringing certain qualities of compassion – for example, empathy, understanding and a commitment to work with our difficulties in a helpful way – we might bring about changes to our struggles in life.	

SECTION II

UNDERSTANDING COMPASSION

We spent some time together in Section I exploring various ways of understanding how and why we can struggle in life. In this next section of the book, we're going to focus on what we can do about this. The origin of the word 'compassion' comes from the Latin words *com*, which means 'with' or 'together', and *pati*, which means 'to bear', or 'to suffer'. So at the heart of the English word 'compassion' is a sense of suffering with or together.

So rather than avoiding, denying or fighting with our difficulties in life, the compassionate mind approach encourages us to meet these directly. We do this through developing various compassionate skills and attributes, and we will explore what these are in the coming chapters of this section. This is all well and good, but what happens if we find the idea of becoming more compassionate with ourselves and others difficult? What if the idea of engaging with our distress seems scary? Or we feel that trying to alleviate distress isn't deserved? Well, in this case it's likely to make working with our own and other people's difficulties much harder. So the final chapter in this section will help us to learn about the types of difficulties we might have in developing our compassionate minds.

5 What is compassion?

'Our human compassion binds us the one to the other – not in pity or patronizingly, but as human beings who have learnt how to turn our common suffering into hope for the future.'

– Nelson Mandela

In the introduction to this book we touched on the importance of understanding what we mean by the term 'compassion'. In this chapter, we're going to look more deeply into the nature of compassion, including:

- Getting a clearer idea on what compassion is and what it is not
- Identifying the key qualities of compassion
- Considering how we can train and strengthen those key qualities of compassion
- Outlining some of the benefits to be gained by this training.

What is compassion?

As we mentioned in the introductory chapter of this workbook, the definition of compassion that we use in Compassionate Mind Training (CMT) is:

'A sensitivity to the suffering of self and others (and its causes), with a commitment to relieve and prevent it.'

So with this definition in mind, let's spend a minute or so thinking about what comes to mind. What does this definition leave you thinking, and feeling?

_____

_____

_____

In CMT, this definition has two different but related psychologies or mindstates:

(i) First Psychology of Compassion – Engagement with distress

This reflects the first line of the above definition – 'sensitivity to the suffering of self and others'. Engagement with distress involves *paying attention to*, as well turning towards distress. This reflects our ability to be aware of and notice suffering, and to move towards it. Given this, the first psychology of compassion also involves a type of strength and courage to engage with distress, rather than avoiding or turning away from it.

Self-reflection: Think about how the first psychology of compassion works for you. How able do you feel to:

Pay attention to your own, or someone else's suffering?

_____

_____

Turn towards, or engage in, your own or someone else's suffering?

_____

_____

Let's think of an example to help us understand this. Imagine that you meet a friend at a café, and they seem quieter and less engaged in the conversation than usual.

What might help you to engage the first psychology of compassion with this friend? What qualities would help you to pay attention and tune in to what they are experiencing?

_____

_____

_____

_____

What might get in the way of your ability to notice or engage with their difficulties? Is there anything that might inhibit this response in you (e.g. feeling tired or annoyed), or make it harder for you to understand why they might be quieter than usual?

_____

_____

_____

In CMT, we suggest that there are six core attributes or qualities that help us with the first psychology of compassion. We depict the different qualities of compassion in Figure 5.1. Whilst these are not the only qualities that compassion may include, together they help us to pay attention to and engage with distress. We will go through each of these qualities, one at a time, and also provide an opportunity for you to think about how each quality relates to you. Some of these qualities might be easier for us to engage in than others, depending on what else we experience at a given time. We will explore this further as we look at each of the qualities.

Figure 5.1: Qualities of the First Psychology of Compassion – Engagement with Distress

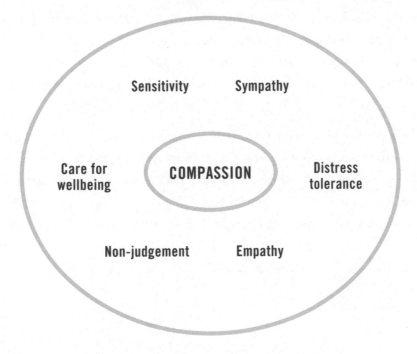

Adapted from Gilbert, *The Compassionate Mind* (2009), reprinted with permission from Constable & Robinson Ltd.

To help explore these qualities, we will use the example of Sarah:

Example: Sarah came to therapy for help with her relationship. She was having frequent arguments with her partner Tanya, and was worried that the relationship was headed for a painful ending. She described how Tanya was working long, unsocial hours, and that she had little energy or interest to do enjoyable things with Sarah as a consequence. In the most recent session she described a particularly bad recent fight in which she had made some cutting and very critical comments about Tanya's personality, after which Tanya had been so upset that she had left the house and stayed with a mutual friend for the night. Sarah was very upset and distressed about this, but also rather angry. She felt that there was nothing she could do to change the situation, and there was 'no hope' of things changing.

Care for wellbeing

A starting point in working with our difficulties in a compassionate way is *motivation*. So rather than ignoring, avoiding or turning away from our difficulties, we try to focus on a part of us that cares about this, that is bothered about our own or others' distress, and wants to work on finding ways to deal with this in a helpful way. Let's look at how this worked for Sarah:

After talking for a while about what was happening in her relationship, Sarah felt less distressed, and was able to reflect a bit more about what was important to her. When asked to focus on the situation from a part of her that was caring and motivated about her own and Tanya's wellbeing, she described that rather than feeling hopeless and resigned, she felt energised. She recognised that she loved Tanya very much, and didn't want to cause her distress. In fact, it was important for her to do what she could to return the relationship to being a source of care, love and happiness.

Self-reflection: How motivated do you feel to try to alleviate someone else's distress and suffering?

_____

_____

How motivated do you typically feel to try and alleviate your distress and suffering?

_____

_____

Are there any things that make it more likely that you will be motivated to engage with distress?

_____

_____

Are there any things that get in the way of this; things that inhibit your ability to be motivated to engage with distress?

_____

_____

Sensitivity

When we are motivated to care, it can be useful to focus our attention on the nature of our pain and distress, so sensitivity here involves learning how to pay attention and tune in to our own (or someone else's) distress. So, rather than blocking out, moving away from or shutting off from difficulties, developing sensitivity allows us to be open to and notice our own (and others') feelings, emotions, thoughts and behaviours.

Helped by her intention to care for her own and Tanya's wellbeing, Sarah was able to direct her attention and notice a number of 'loops in the mind' that were adding extra distress to a situation that was already painful. She noticed that she often became caught up in ruminating about the arguments and things that Tanya had done that left her feeling angry and resentful. She also noticed worry-anxiety based loops linked with concerns that the relationship was 'doomed' and in particular, worries that she would never find anyone else if the relationship ended. Sarah found it helpful to recognise when these loops were whirling through her mind and to see that these were making it more likely that she and Tanya would argue. Crucially, she also found that these loops in her mind (especially angry ruminations) made it harder for her to tune in to how upset and distressed Tanya was feeling about the recent changes in their relationship.

Self-reflection: How able do you feel to be sensitive to other people's distress and suffering? Are you able to tune in to it and be attentive to their feelings, emotions, thoughts and behaviours?

_____

_____

_____

How able do you feel to be sensitive to your own distress and suffering? Are you able to tune in to it and be attentive to your feelings, emotions, thoughts and behaviours?

_____

_____

_____

What helps you to be sensitive to distress?

_____

_____

_____

What gets in the way of you being sensitive to your own, or someone else's, distress?

_____

_____

Sympathy

Sometimes when we think about sympathy, it brings negative connotations to mind, such as pity. However, what we mean by sympathy in CMT is being *emotionally moved* by our own, or other people's distress. You might well have had a sympathetic reaction without realising it. For example, maybe you've seen someone stub their toe, or get their hand trapped in a door, and automatically felt a flush of pain (that 'ow!' moment) yourself. Or perhaps you've been watching someone on TV suffering, or grieving after the loss of a loved one, and found a tear in your eye. So being able to be emotionally moved by other people's pain and distress is important, particularly as it can be a precursor to trying to do something to alleviate the suffering. Having sympathy for yourself involves a similar process – being emotionally open to your own pain is an important step towards having compassion for yourself – *self-compassion*.

> Having tuned in to her own 'loops in the mind', Sarah began to get in contact with a new set of feelings. She started to feel a sense of sadness at how things had changed for her and Tanya, and about how much pain they'd both been in without being able to do anything helpful. Unlike her initial distress, she felt more moved by Tanya's distress – that she had been working hard to pay the bills so that both of them could live a life they wanted to.

Self-reflection: How easy is it for you to engage in sympathy, and the emotions/feelings that can go with this? Can you be emotionally open to, and moved by, other people's suffering?

_____

_____

Can you be emotionally open to, and moved by, your own suffering?

_____

_____

What helps you to feel moved by your own, or someone else's, distress?

_____

_____

What gets in the way of you being emotionally moved by your own, or someone else's, distress?

_____

_____

Distress tolerance

As you might imagine, developing motivation to care for oneself, becoming more sensitive to suffering and being emotionally moved by distress (sympathy) might sound helpful on paper, but they are qualities also likely to bring us into contact with some quite difficult and potentially painful feelings. Given this, it is important that we learn to tolerate this distress, or develop _distress tolerance_. This involves learning that distress and painful feelings pass; that like a wave we can 'ride' difficult emotions and remain grounded and stable in the presence of them. Bearing and tolerating distress in this way makes it possible for us to do something about it. If we're unable to open our hearts to and remain tolerant of pain it is likely to be hard to engage with our difficulties (or those of other people), and find ways to address them.

> Partly by focusing on her motivation to care for her own and Tanya's wellbeing, as well as her emotional connection to Tanya's pain, Sarah felt that it was important to also work on remaining grounded and strong during these times of difficulty. She 'set' herself the intention of practising tolerating her distress, sadness and anger

towards Tanya and the relationship. Sarah recognised that if she could tolerate these feelings, she was more likely to achieve what she really wanted – closeness, connection and happiness with Tanya.

Self-reflection: How able do you feel to compassionately tolerate other people's pain and distress? To accept and be with it, without feeling resigned, defeated, overwhelmed, or powerless.

_____

_____

How able do you feel to compassionately tolerate your own pain and distress? To accept and to be able to be with it, without feeling resigned, defeated, overwhelmed, or powerless.

_____

_____

What makes it easier to be able to tolerate your own – or someone else's – distress and suffering?

_____

_____

What makes it harder, or blocks you from, tolerating your own or someone else's distress?

_____

_____

Empathy

Empathy involves a variety of qualities; being emotionally in tune with someone (feeling 'with' them) but being able to imagine the experiences of others, and to be aware of why they might be feeling, thinking or behaving in the way that they are. So one aspect of empathy is to look at what sits behind someone's behaviour or response, considering what might have led them to act in a particular way (e.g. their emotions or motives), rather than just focusing on the response itself. Unlike sympathy, which is automatic 'feeling with', empathy takes effort and practice to take a different perspective from that of your own. Often this can involve trying to imagine what it would be like to be in the shoes of the other. This can lead to considering what would be helpful for the other person, given our understanding of what has led them to feel as they do. Whilst we have traditionally considered empathy as directed at others, we can also think about how we might have empathy for ourselves; that is, how we can bring a certain understanding and perspective-taking to our own minds, emotions, and responses, and consider what might be helpful for us given that understanding.

> Sarah found that once she felt more confident in tolerating her distress, it was easier to bring empathy to the situation. She was able to see what sat behind many of the arguments they were having – stress, worry and a lack of quality time together. She began to understand – almost as if looking from a different vantage point – how and why the arguments had happened, and how in many ways, they were an expression of pain both she and Tanya were experiencing.

Self-reflection: Think about your capacity to bring an empathic stance to other people's difficulties, and what has led to them?

_____

_____

_____

Think about your capacity to bring an empathic stance to your own difficulties. Can you understand and take a compassionate perspective of the nature of your difficulties, and what has led to them?

_____

_____

_____

What helps you to have empathy for yourself or others?

_____

_____

What blocks or makes it harder for you to have empathy for yourself or someone else?

_____

_____

Non-judgement

As we've explored in earlier chapters, we have tricky brains, and at times these can lead us – and other people – to behave in ways that can be difficult to understand. At these times, we can criticise others and ourselves for what has happened. This in turn tends to exacerbate our struggles and blocks helpful action. The quality of compassionate non-judgement involves trying to step back from judging, criticising or condemning the complexities of our own or other people's minds. It involves an acceptance of the difficult things that our complex minds can bring to the world and our relationships – for example, volatile emotions, aggression and hostility, and even cruelty.

Non-judgement does not mean you don't have preferences, become passive, complacent or excusing/accepting of unpleasant behaviour. Rather, in compassionate non-judgement, we try to step back from our threat minds – and in particular our capacity for (self-) criticism and condemnation – so that we have a chance to clearly see into the nature of our own and others' difficulties, have greater perspective and reflect on what might be helpful. As Carl Jung, former student of Sigmund Freud and an eminent psychologist himself, said: 'Thinking is difficult, that's why most people judge.'

Sarah recognised that she had been very judgemental over the past month or two. She described how given the frequency of their arguments she would often feel quite critical and condemning of Tanya, and judgemental about their relationship. However, she found that having a greater empathy for why they had been getting caught up in this was helpful in allowing her to step back from judging. She was still bothered about how many arguments they were having, but recognised that arguments could also be a normal part of healthy relationships, and that her judgements and hostility about Tanya and the arguments were only adding to the difficulties both of them were experiencing.

Self-reflection: Think about how often you judge yourself and others. Are you able to step back from this and try to take a non-judgemental stance?

_____

_____

_____

What helps you to take a non-judging stance with yourself or others?

_____

_____

What blocks or hinders your ability to be non-judging with yourself or others?

_____

_____

Summary

In this section we have explored the six core attributes or qualities that, in conjunction, help to give rise to the first psychology of compassion – the ability and intention to engage and be sensitive to suffering. We're now going to explore the skills that can give rise to the second psychology of compassion.

Second Psychology of Compassion – Alleviation of Distress

The second psychology of compassion involves a desire to acquire the skills and wisdom to try and do something about suffering – to find the courage and understanding (wisdom) to alleviate it and prevent it from returning. Let's think about an example of this. Imagine that you want to be a doctor, and are focused on caring and helping people who are ill and in pain. This would be an example of your intention (i.e. to help people), and it would almost certainly help if you were also caring and sensitive to others' distress (so, the first psychology of compassion). However, you would also need to study for many years to develop the skills and knowledge of how best to do this. So intention here is not enough on its own. From a CMT perspective, it's also important to apply this when considering our own difficulties and distress. Intention to engage with and do something about our difficulties is important, but we also need to have the wisdom, strength and skills to be able to do so.

Self-reflection: Think about the second psychology of compassion. How able do you feel to alleviate your own, or someone else's, suffering? Do you feel that you have the skills, wisdom and strength to do this?

_____

_____

What helps you to try and alleviate your own, or someone else's, suffering? What makes this harder?

_____

_____

_____

_____

Don't worry at this stage if you don't feel you have the skills or knowledge to be able to alleviate your difficulties – that's what we're going to come to in Sections III, IV and V. However, before we get to developing skills, it might be useful for us to briefly outline what these skills are, and how developing them will help to build your compassionate mind.

There are a variety of ways to help you develop skills in the second psychology of compassion. This is depicted in Figure 5.2 below. Those keen-eyed readers may recognise the inner circle in this diagram as the attributes that we discussed earlier in the chapter. The outer circle shows the different skills we will practise in this book that can help to 'tone up', like a muscle, our compassionate mind attributes (shown in the inner circle).

Figure 5.2: The compassion circles – the key attributes of compassion
(first psychology – inner circle) and the skills to develop them
(second psychology – outer circle)

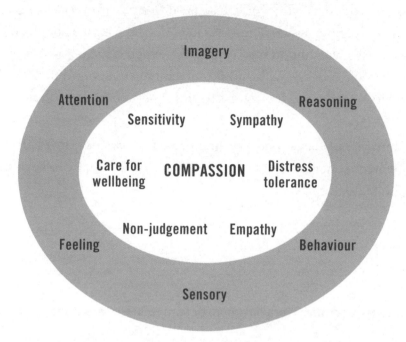

From Gilbert, *The Compassionate Mind* (2009), reprinted with permission from
Constable & Robinson Ltd.

Skills training – The Second Psychology of Compassion

Looking at the outer circle of Figure 5.2 above, we can see there are six key areas of skill training that can be used as the second psychology of compassion. We will outline these below, and return to the example of Sarah to help us with this.

Compassionate attention: Many of us can get caught up focusing on things that trigger, maintain or even exacerbate our threat systems and distress. At times we might not even realise that this is happening. So developing skills in compassionate attention involves learning to focus on things that are helpful and useful to us. Imagine that you go on a date, which overall goes really well, but at one point you share a story that you think is humorous, only for your date to not find it funny. After the date, you find your attention locked in to focusing on this one negative moment, rather than the other three hours of great conversation and fun. So here compassionate attention may be about noticing where your attention is being dragged to, and practising gently shifting this to parts of the date that went really well, or to other things that are helpful (for example, the fact that your date has texted to ask you to go out again later in the week).

Some of these skills are referred to as mindfulness, which has been described as 'paying attention, in the present moment, without judgement'. We will explore how to develop and practise mindfulness in Chapter 8 (pages 101–119).

> Sarah liked the idea of learning how to become more aware and mindful. She started to practise outside of sessions, and was pleased when she began to notice when her threat system was activated. In moments when she found herself worrying that nothing would ever change in the relationship, she also described being able to broaden the scope – to focus on things that had been going well between her and Tanya, and situations that she felt she'd handled well.

Compassionate imagery: Our ability to use our new brain competency to imagine and fantasise about things is a powerful tool that CMT makes use of. A key aspect of imagery is that what we imagine can actually produce similar physiological responses in our body to 'real' experiences. So for example, seeing someone we find sexually attractive, and imagining that same person (when they are not present), can create the same physiological response in our bodies (e.g. arousal). We will explore this in more detail in Chapter 10. Key at this point, however, is to hold in mind that we can use imagery to help create compassion-specific images, and to develop our compassionate minds.

> Sarah used her imagination to picture how she would respond to difficult situations in the future. She imagined a version of her that was more grounded, patient and understanding, and how that part would react to Tanya.

We will explore how we can train and develop imagery skills in Chapters 10–17.

Compassionate reasoning and thinking: Many of us can get caught up in threat-based thinking patterns linked to worrying about the future, ruminating about things from the past, and self-criticism about aspects of ourselves (e.g. our behaviour, identity, appearance and so forth). Compassionate reasoning and thinking involves training our minds so that we can deliberately engage in more helpful, caring and compassionate ways of thinking about ourselves, other people and situations we find ourselves in. This might involve guiding our thinking – for example, asking ourselves, 'What might be a helpful way to think about this difficulty/situation?' Or, we could consider what we might say to a loved one if they were going through the difficulty we are experiencing.

> Sarah took some time to write out helpful ways in which she could think about her recent difficulties. She recognised that rather than taking the difficulties to mean that the relationship was hopeless, she could see these difficulties as an opportunity to learn how to act and respond differently in her relationship. She was also able to voice some self-compassionate thoughts of understanding – that this had been a difficult time for her, and that, given her previous difficult relationship it was not surprising that she might be sensitive to the difficulties she and Tanya had been having.

We will return to look at how we can develop compassionate thinking in Chapter 19.

Compassionate behaviour: The way we behave and act in the world can have important benefits for how we feel, and can impact on our relationships. Compassionate behaviour is not just 'being nice' or 'being kind' (although of course, sometimes it might be) and it is important to separate out genuine compassion from submissive compassion, which is linked to trying to behave in ways so that others will like us or not reject us. Genuine compassionate behaviours involve working out (with wisdom) the actions and behaviours that help us to alleviate our own, or someone else's, distress and suffering – that help us to develop, grow and flourish. At times this may be learning how to be assertive and to say 'no'. Key to compassionate behaviour is having the strength and courage to approach and engage with the things that are difficult. There are, of course, different types of compassionate behaviours, and those that are important or useful in the short term ('What might be the most helpful thing I can do today/tomorrow/this week?') may be different to those that would get us to a better place in the long term. We may engage in a short-term behaviour that could be helpful, such as seeing a friend or going for a massage, or responding to a difficult text message or email, rather than avoiding it. We may also decide to commit to longer-term actions, such as practising compassionate mind training exercises each day for ten minutes.

> Sarah was very clear about what she wanted to do. Rather than avoid talking about their problems, she decided to organise a time to speak to Tanya about what had been happening, but to do this at a time when she was more likely to be heard and when they would have a positive outcome (e.g. not late at night after Tanya had just finished a long day at work). She also decided that she would practise mindfulness and breathing exercises for five minutes every day over the next month.

We will return to how to train and develop our compassionate behaviours in Chapter 21.

Compassionate sensory focusing: Taking a sensory focus involves stimulating our different senses (e.g. smell, hearing, touch) within a broad body focus, which can help to stimulate affiliative positive emotion and more broadly, the conditions for compassion. There is a lot of scientific evidence suggesting that bringing a sensory and bodily focus can be helpful in regulating our distress (e.g. by stimulating our soothing system). Therefore learning how to breathe in ways that help the body slow down, or adopting certain body postures may help us to feel more grounded, balanced and strong.

> Although Sarah was feeling more confident about finding a positive outcome to her recent difficulties, she recognised that these steps were likely to be difficult in themselves. To help herself to remain grounded and balanced, she decided to rejoin her yoga course, and to practise a number of breathing exercises to help her slow down and tolerate stress.

We will explore a sensory focus in Chapters 9 and 10, and also throughout many parts of this book.

Compassionate feelings: In recent years, scientists have found that practising and developing our positive emotions can have a powerful impact on our ability to tolerate and reduce our distress, as well as to enhance our wellbeing and help us flourish. This has also been the focus of many practices within Buddhist traditions. In CMT we spend time generating and practising certain positive emotions linked to compassion, including the wish that oneself and others are free of suffering, and experience happiness. These feelings include warmth, kindness, friendliness and contentment.

> It was not hard for Sarah to realise that in recent months she had been connected with a lot of powerful negative emotions (anger, anxiety and sadness). Although she felt more able to work with these, she described missing positive emotions in her life. She decided that it would be helpful if she could re-connect with these feelings through seeing friends and engaging in activities that she previously enjoyed, such as playing netball, meeting friends for food, and watching movies. She also decided to spend time practising exercises that helped to enhance the emotions of the drive and soothing systems.

We will explore how to develop these types of positive feelings in Chapters 9, 10 and 11.

Bringing it all together

When we look at the six aspects of how to engage with our suffering and our difficulties, and then look at the six aspects of how we can help ourselves and others, this can seem a bit overwhelming at first. A good comparison here may be to remember when you first learnt to drive a car: you had to keep in mind the accelerator and brake pedals, whilst working out how to change gears, use indictors and mirrors. And of course, most importantly, you needed to steer and avoid hitting other cars, lampposts and people! However, with practice, gradually it all came together, and became a whole lot easier to coordinate these tasks and skills in an integrated way. It is the same with compassion – it looks tricky to start with but as you get the hang of it, it all falls into place. Remember, at its core compassion involves two key things: learning how we can be sensitive and engage with our own/others' suffering and difficulties, and how we can use our skills (wisdom) to try and work out what might be the most useful way to help.

Over time, it can be helpful to think about practising these attributes and skills as a type of mind training. Each time we engage in them, we are triggering particular networks of brain cells (called neurons) and physiological experiences in our body. Just like working out in the gym, the more we practise these, the stronger they are likely to become, and the more likely we are to be able to use them in a helpful way when needed in the future (i.e. when we are distressed). These compassion 'patterns' are only one such pattern. We could have the same for an angry, anxious and self-critical way of being. So our intention here – and what we will help you to practise in the coming sections of the book – is to support you in training yourself in 'being' this compassionate pattern, your 'compassionate mind' or the 'compassionate version' of yourself, as often as possible.

We will return to these ideas – and help you to learn more about how we can develop and direct our compassionate minds – in Sections III and IV.

Hints and tips: Difficulties with the two psychologies

Try not to worry if you find it difficult to do one (or both) of the two psychologies of compassion. There will be times when we may all find aspects of these difficult, but it may be helpful to take a look at Box 5.1 below to see some of the reasons people sometimes struggle with these.

Box 5.1: Some common difficulties with the two psychologies

Common difficulties	Helpful hints
First Psychology Difficulties I feel confident in some of the attributes, but not in all of them.	This is quite common. Try not to worry about this too much at this stage. Maybe you can check back in with these as you progress through this book and develop your compassionate mind.
I can be caring, sensitive and empathic to other people's distress at times, but only if their distress isn't too strong.	As we begin to develop our compassionate minds, we will learn how to develop skills that will help us to manage these types of difficulties. We'll also see that a core quality of compassion is developing strength and courage to help us to tolerate distress.
Do I have to be able to do all six of these attributes to be sensitive to and to engage in my own or someone else's suffering?	Not necessarily. There may be times when you feel more confident in some of these than others, and will still be able to engage well in the first psychology of compassion. But overall, these attributes tend to support each other – so, for example, if we are able to have strength and tolerate distress, this supports us in being sensitive and motivated to engage in suffering. If we can connect with non-judgement, this helps us to have empathy for our own or others' distress.
Second Psychology Difficulties I think I have some qualities of compassion, but I don't feel very confident in finding ways to alleviate my difficulties.	That's OK, we'll be helping you to learn how to develop your skills in Sections III and IV of this book.
There seem to be a lot of different things I have to think about and learn in order for me to develop a compassionate mind – it's putting me off a bit.	Just as when we start learning many things for the first time (for example, a new language or a musical instrument) it can initially feel a bit overwhelming. But as with other things, taking small steps and encouraging yourself to do what you can is helpful. Do take things in your own time and remember, we'll help you through this book in a step-by-step way.

Of course, the type of struggles described above can come and go – sometimes they might feel stronger, other times less prominent. And some people may struggle with both psychologies at the same time, which can complicate the picture. But we will go on to help you work with these in the coming sections of the book.

Chapter summary

In this chapter we've taken a closer look at the way we understand and develop compassion in Compassionate Mind Training (CMT), including the different qualities and skills that allow us to engage with distress and find ways to alleviate it.

What we have learnt together	My personal reflections on the chapter
In this chapter we have explored: 1. The definition of compassion as involving two psychologies – a sensitivity to suffering, and a desire to alleviate and prevent suffering. 2. That there are different qualities or attributes of compassion – care for wellbeing, sensitivity, sympathy, distress tolerance, empathy and non-judgement. 3. That there can be things that can block or inhibit our compassionate qualities, and things that can support or facilitate them. 4. That there are a variety of skills that help form the second psychology of compassion – attention, thinking and reasoning, emotion, behaviour, sensory focus and imagery. 5. That through developing and applying the different attributes and skills of compassion, we can find ways to engage with our difficulties and work towards bringing about helpful change.	

6 The three flows of compassion

'If you want others to be happy, practise compassion. If you want to be happy, practise compassion.'

– Dalai Lama, The Art of Happiness (1998)

When asked about compassion, most people's initial thoughts relate to how this is directed *towards* someone else. We are often compassionate to those we love and care for – our family, children, friends, neighbours and colleagues. However, this is only one of the three possible 'flows' that compassion can be directed towards. Not only can we direct compassion towards others, but we can also experience compassion flowing from others towards us, as well as direct compassion to ourselves. Although these three flows have overlaps between them, they are not simply the same thing. In fact, it may well be that we need different skills – and face different challenges – in practising and experiencing each of these. We will explore these in turn below.

1. Compassion for others

Compassion for others involves us being aware of and sensitive to the suffering in others, being able to move towards or engage with it, and having the desire to try and alleviate it. For example, seeing someone who has fallen and in pain, and trying to help them in some way, maybe by comforting them, helping them up, or taking them to see a doctor. Studies suggest that developing and expressing compassion for others has a variety of benefits for the person that we're being compassionate to. However, we also know that the brain and body systems that are stimulated when we're being compassionate to others have positive effects on us too.

Self-reflection: How able do you feel to direct compassion towards other people?

_____

_____

Are there certain things that make it easier for you to direct care and compassion to others?

_____

_____

We will explore how to direct and develop compassion to others in Chapter 15.

2. Compassion from others

Being open to the care, kindness and support of others can be a very powerful experience. You might be able to think about a time when you experienced this. For many of us, others' compassion can produce a reassuring or calming effect in us, sometimes even reducing the level of our distress or pain. Research studies have shown that experiencing care and kindness from others can have powerful physiological effects upon our brains and bodies, and a major impact on regulating our threat system. In fact, if you think about it, we are set up to receive compassion from a very early age. Take a distressed baby, for example. Their crying – whether because they are hungry or in need of contact and warmth – signals this to their parent, who notices and sensitively turns towards this distress, and then engages in behaviours that might help to alleviate this. In fact, throughout our childhood, adolescence and even in adulthood, the care and compassion of others has a significant effect in helping us manage our difficulties. This can range from the sensitivity, encouragement and reassurance that our parents give us the first day we leave on our own for school, to the empathy and support from a friend when we first have our heart broken, or when we experience a bereavement. In all of these situations having someone who is sensitive, caring and supportive can help us to feel held and empowered, and less distressed, overwhelmed and alone.

Self-reflection: Take a moment to think about the times in life when you have received care or compassion from others. How able were/are you to receive compassion and care from other people?

_____

_____

Are there certain things that make it easier for you to experience care and compassion from others?

_____

_____

We will help you to find ways of practising experiencing compassion from others in Chapter 16.

3. Compassion for oneself (self-compassion)

The final flow of compassion is often the most difficult for us – directing compassion to ourselves, commonly known as self-compassion. In self-compassion, we try to become sensitive to the nature of our own pain, to find ways to engage with it, and then develop the skills and motivation to alleviate this. There are different ways of thinking about this: one is to consider how you might think, feel or behave towards yourself, in the way that a really caring friend or family member would treat you if you were distressed. Alternatively, you could consider how you might apply to yourself the same compassionate way of responding to loved others who are distressed.

Self-reflection: How able do you feel to direct compassion towards yourself?

_____

_____

Are there certain things that make it easier to be compassionate to yourself?

_____

_____

It can be helpful to find ways of cultivating compassion for ourselves, and we will look at this in more detail in Chapter 17, and throughout Section V.

Self-reflection: Think about the three flows of compassion outlined above. Which of these do you find easier? Which are more difficult?

_____

_____

_____

_____

Chapter summary

We've continued to develop our understanding of compassion in this chapter by exploring how compassion can be directed in three different ways, each of which can have important effects upon our brains and bodies, and in particular, our emotions, how we manage difficulties, and ultimately, our wellbeing.

What we have learnt together	My personal reflections on the chapter
In this chapter, we explored: 1. The three different 'flows' of compassion. These are: • Giving compassion to others • Receiving compassion from others • Giving compassion to ourselves (self-compassion).	

2.   We also reflected on whether any of these flows are easier or more difficult for us, and thought about what experiences might block or facilitate the flow of compassion.

7 Why compassion can be difficult

'The heart is like a garden. It can grow compassion or fear, resentment or love. What seeds will you plant there?'

Jack Kornfield, Buddha's Little Instruction Book (1996)

In the previous chapters we have spent some time exploring compassion in detail, including ideas around its two psychologies of turning towards, engaging and working with suffering and difficulties in ourselves and others, and then working out how best to try to alleviate these. We noted these competencies can be used if you are being compassionate to other people, if you are open to others being compassionate to you, and if you are being compassionate with your own life difficulties.

During this exploration we have also begun to touch on potential difficulties with directing our minds to compassion. Whilst many of us are encouraged to be kind and compassionate to other people, we're not always taught how to do this or how to work through difficulties that are common in doing this. It is even less common for us to be taught how we can be compassionate towards ourselves, or why we can struggle to engage in this way of treating ourselves, even if we can do it for others. It turns out that compassion can be tricky for a number of reasons, and we're therefore going to spend time in this chapter exploring why this might be, and what we can do if this is the case.

Why we find compassion hard: The fears, blocks and resistances to compassion

In Compassionate Mind Training (CMT) we refer to the difficulties we can have with compassion as FBRs – the fears, blocks and resistances to compassion. *Fears* of compassion are when we would like to be compassionate but we're frightened of the feelings that arise when we try or worry about what might happen to us if we do become more compassionate. We might be frightened we will become weak in some way or overly sensitive. As Carl Jung said:

'The most terrifying thing is to accept oneself completely' and when it comes to cultivating compassion, particularly compassion for yourself, this is certainly a common experience for many people that we've worked with. For some, connecting with compassion is scary as it may open them up to other emotions that may worry or overwhelm them. Here are a couple of examples:

Example: Jane had a very difficult upbringing, with little care or affection, and her parents often treated her with criticism and hostility. In therapy, she didn't like the idea of compassion for herself. After exploration with her therapist, she was able to connect this to a fear that if she was to become compassionate to herself and her early experiences, this would mean that she would get in contact with a lot of anger or rage that she had been holding onto from her childhood, that had not been safe to express.

Example: David had an initially caring and loving relationship with his parents until his mother died from breast cancer and his father became very depressed. David's difficulty with experiencing compassion from others as an adult turned out to be linked to his fear of beginning to trust that others would be there, and then them disappearing. He was also able to describe feeling scared about receiving care and compassion from other people. He was also concerned that receiving care and compassion from others would connect him to memories of bereavement from the past and powerful feelings of sadness and grief that he had never learned how to deal with.

Blocks are things that arise when people would like to be compassionate and are not frightened of it, but find that things seem to get in the way of this happening. They might describe being too busy in life to dedicate time to practising their compassionate mind skills – for example, they may have many other competing demands on their time (e.g. the gym, seeing friends and family). For others, it may be that circumstances prevent them from practising compassion (for example, many nurses, doctors and other people in the 'caring' professions often complain they would like to be more compassionate with their patients but have too much paperwork to allow them to do this).

Resistances are when we are not frightened or blocked to compassion, but we simply don't want to engage in it. For example, we might not want to be compassionate to our worst enemy, to someone we do not feel deserves it (i.e. they 'brought their difficulties on themselves'). We may also resist being compassionate to ourselves for something we feel ashamed of – a sort of 'I don't deserve compassion' way of thinking.

Of course, it might be that fears, blocks and resistances blend into each other. For example, it might be that a resistance actually turns out to be linked more to an underlying fear. Regardless, here are some other common difficulties that people have with compassion:

- *Self-monitoring and self-criticism:* If we're really caught up with our threat system this can block or stop us from focusing on other things, such as compassion. So, just as clouds in the sky block the sun, our evolved capacity to self-monitor, and in particular, get caught up in a pattern of self-monitoring and self-criticism (that may be fuelled by powerful negative emotions such as anger or disgust towards self), can prevent us from being able to be compassionate and caring towards ourselves and others.

- *Compassion as 'weak':* Often when the word 'compassion' is mentioned in the CMT groups we run, a common response is – 'I don't like it, it's weak' or 'I don't like the sound of that, it'll make me vulnerable'. Here, there are beliefs – often learnt over a period of many years – that being compassionate to others makes you vulnerable, weak and able to be taken advantage of or hurt.

- *Compassion as letting ourselves off the hook:* For many people, being compassionate towards ourselves (or others) would mean letting ourselves (or others) off the hook, or allowing ourselves to get away with mistakes or even making excuses. For example, Clive came to therapy feeling depressed and self-critical after the break-up of his marriage. His wife had found out about an affair he had been having for six months and left him. Clive described wanting to resist becoming compassionate for the struggles he was experiencing, fearing that if he were to, he would no longer care about the mistakes he had made in the past, and might be more likely to make them again in the future.

- *Compassion as 'alien':* Whilst compassion is linked to the innate motivation we have as a mammal to be caring to others, it is not guaranteed that we will all be able to direct or receive it. Research suggests that unless we have the lived experiences that have allowed us to learn compassion – how to express it, how to receive it – it may feel quite alien and uncomfortable for us, a little like trying to speak a foreign language for the first time. But just as we can all learn a new language over time (although for some of us – both of us included! – this can be difficult), so we can with compassion, even if this isn't something that you know about or feel confident with yet.

- *Painful memories:* Sadly, some of us will have very unpleasant or scary experiences in life. Sometimes these are things related to events – for example, a car crash or accident of some type. However, a particularly difficult type of trauma for humans – especially when we are thinking about compassion – is trauma that has come at the hands of other people. This type of *relational* trauma – whether in a verbal, physical or sexual manner – is often referred to as abuse. This proves to be a particularly powerful experience that can block our capacity to connect with compassion later in life; in a sense, we learn that rather than being sources of compassion, care and kindness, other people can be, and have been, the source of threat and suffering. We will return to this in Chapter xx. It may also be that you would also find our colleague Deborah Lee's book, *The Compassionate Mind Approach to Recovering From Trauma*, helpful with this as well.

Self-reflection: Having read through some of the common difficulties with compassion above, do any of them sound familiar? What fears, blocks or resistances to compassion are you aware of?

Can you think of reasons why you might have some of these fears or blocks to compassion? Does it make sense that this might be the case?

If you're interested in learning more about your own fears or blocks to compassion, you might be like to complete the 'Fears of Compassion' questionnaire that Paul Gilbert and his colleagues developed. You can find a copy of this online: www.compassionatemind.co.uk.

When you complete this questionnaire you can simply add up the scores for each of the three subscales. This might give you an idea if one of the 'flows' of compassion is trickier for you than another. You might also find it interesting to look through each of the three subscales and see which – if any – items you tended to endorse the highest. This might also give you an idea about what specific fears or concerns could lay behind your struggle to develop compassion. Some of the research looking at fears of compassion has found that these concerns are related to higher levels of mental health symptomology, but also to a general fear of happiness.

Try not to worry if your scores come out higher than you expected, or if you find the idea of compassion is quite scary. This book is designed to help you work through these difficulties, and we'll return to this throughout the coming sections of the workbook. Like many other fears in life though, taking small steps towards these, slowly and gradually building up our distress tolerance, understanding and courage, usually helps the fears to lose some of the power over us. We've also dedicated Chapter 25 to help with this specifically.

Chapter summary

Although we've been learning in this section about the meaning, definition and qualities of compassion, in this chapter we've focused more closely on how we can actually find compassion quite difficult.

What we have learnt together	My personal reflections on the chapter
1. That whilst many people find compassion helpful, for others, this can trigger a variety of difficulties.	
2. That there are various fears, blocks and resistances to compassion.	
3. That these difficulties with compassion often make sense, given our experiences in life.	
4. That we will return to how we can help you to work with your fears, blocks or resistances to compassion later in the workbook.	

SECTION III

BUILDING CAPACITY:
Developing the Foundations for Our Compassionate Mind

In the following chapters, we will help you to start the process of developing your compassionate mind. To begin with, it can be helpful to spend some time together creating a sound base for this. Just as you would lay good foundations before building a house, it is also helpful to build skills that help 'prepare' the compassionate mind. To do this, we will help you to:

• Develop your skills of compassionate attention, awareness and mindfulness

• Develop your soothing system (through breathing practices, voice tones, body posture and imagery)

• Develop a healthy and balanced drive system.

Is it possible to change our brains?

In recent years, scientists have learned much more about how our brains work. One particularly interesting finding has been that our brains are actually far more plastic than previously thought. Now, of course this doesn't mean they're made of the material plastic! Instead, it refers to how the connections between the cells in our brain (called neurons) have an amazing ability to reorganise themselves into different patterns. So, like the way our bodies can change shape depending on whether we exercise or eat too much food, so too can our brains.

For some of us, certain patterns in the brain – for example, those for self-criticism or worry – might be getting too much of a workout. So it might be helpful to practise new sets of brain patterns that, rather than stimulating and strengthening the threat system, may help us to reduce the activation of this system and instead help to develop and strengthen our soothing and drive systems.

How to practise

We have written the following chapters to form a step-by-step process of skill practice and development, so that one can build on another. However, different people find some of the coming exercises easier than others, so try not to worry too much – or to be too hard on yourself – if you find some parts more difficult than others. We'll guide you in things that can help navigate these difficulties and find ways to support your practice.

As with exercise, it's helpful if we can do a little bit of practice on a regular basis. Now, each person finds their own way with this, but, to start with, if you can allocate five to ten minutes each day to practise some of the coming exercises, that would be great, and likely to help you on your journey to developing your compassionate mind. However, if this amount of practice isn't possible, remember that like exercise, doing some practice is better than none. Of course, if you feel able to do more than ten minutes, that would be great too. You may not notice any changes to start with, and it can be quite easy to start thinking 'This isn't going to work, I'm just going to give up' and lose faith in continuing your efforts. Whilst this disappointment is understandable, if we can tap in to our wisdom and understanding about how change happens – and in particular, the pace at which change happens – that can help us when we're starting our practice. If you remember back to Chapter 5 and the compassion circles (see page 82), an important starting place for compassion is motivation and desire, and this might be helpful to remind yourself of throughout the coming chapters: 'I'm spending time practising this because it's important for me to learn more about my difficulties in life, and to find ways to do something helpful about them.'

8 Attention and mindfulness

'Your vision will become clear only when you look into your heart. Who looks outside, dreams. Who looks inside, awakens.'

– Carl Jung

As we've explored so far in this workbook, we can all be vulnerable to our threat systems grabbing hold of our attention. We can struggle with anxious thoughts about the future, or ruminate about mistakes we've made in the past. We can criticise ourselves in all sorts of ways. Sometimes when this happens it can feel like our awareness is captured and held hostage to what our threat system wants it to focus on, rather than what we would like it to focus on. In some ways it can feel like the dog is walking us, rather than the other way round! This experience, and our struggle against it, can cause us lots of stress and suffering. However, there are steps that we can take – and skills we can develop – to help with this. One of these skills is called *mindfulness*.

Mindfulness

There are many ways we can develop our skills in compassion, and a crucial one is mindfulness. There have been a number of attempts to describe what mindfulness is. At its heart, mindfulness involves learning to pay attention in the present moment, without judgement or evaluation. The process therefore involves a combination of directing attention in a particular way – to the present moment – and an *intention* to do this without engaging in our tendency to judge or criticise what we are paying attention to. In this sense mindfulness involves consciously being aware of and observing our experiences – again and again and again.

As we strengthen our mindfulness skills we may develop our awareness and observation in a way that allows us *to know what we're experiencing, while we're experiencing it*. In turn, this can help us to notice and become curious of the nature of our mind and its natural tendency to be tricky. For example, we can notice how our minds tend to hop around and get caught up in certain patterns (e.g. new brain – old brain loops which we explored in Chapter 1, see pages 3–15). If we are unable to notice and recognise what is happening – and how this is contributing to our difficulties and distress – it's likely to be difficult for us to do anything effective to help ourselves. Throughout the rest of this chapter, we will help you to practise ways of training your attention so that you are able to notice, and then step out of, these loops in the mind. We will start by focusing on different aspects of attention itself.

Understanding attention

Attention is often understood as a mental ability that involves a form of 'noticing'. Key to this is that attention can be *consciously directed*, and depending on what it is directed to, it can have a powerful effect on our feelings. One way of thinking about attention is by comparing it to a spotlight; that is, like a spotlight, it can be moved around and 'shone' in different directions. Just as a spotlight lights up what it shines on, when we focus our attention on something, this can also light up our physiology and feelings. Let's consider an example. Spend a moment directing your attention to a memory of a recent time when you felt angry about something. This could have been an argument you had with someone, or maybe something you saw on the news or read in the paper. Spend fifteen to thirty seconds really focusing your attention back on this.

Self-reflection: How did focusing on this memory leave you feeling? _____

_____

Now let's focus your attention on a time in your life when you felt really, really happy. Maybe a time when you were with friends or family, received a compliment or good news, or were connected with nature. Spend fifteen to thirty seconds directing your attention to this.

Self-reflection: How did focusing on this memory leave you feeling? _____

_____

What you might have noticed from these brief, directed attention exercises is that not only were you able to direct your attention to something specific (a memory), but that doing so may have triggered a similar type of feeling or emotion that you had at the time. Here's another way of exploring the nature and power of our attention.

Exercise – learning about attention

Let's try a short exercise. For this, find a comfortable place to sit for a few minutes. To start with, try and place all of your attention on your left foot. Spend fifteen seconds or so really paying attention to whatever sensations you can notice in this part of your body. If it helps, wiggle the toes of your left foot. After fifteen seconds, move your attention to your right foot – try and pay attention to the sensations located in your right foot. Again, if it helps, wiggle the toes of your right foot, noticing as much as you can do. Now move your attention to your left hand. Pay attention to whatever sensations are present in this area of your body. If it helps, rub together your thumb and fingers of your left hand. Again, just notice the sensation present. Again, after fifteen seconds or so, shift your attention to your right hand and again, rub together the thumb and fingers of your right hand, paying attention to whatever sensation is present there. Finally, shift your attention to your face. Try and notice any sensations that are present there. Move or maybe lick your lips, again just noticing whatever sensations are present as you do this.

Self-reflection: What did you make of this exercise? What learning points can you take from it?

_____

_____

_____

_____

Although people take different things from this exercise, the following are some common, and important, observations about the nature of our attention:

- Our attention can be consciously directed – it is 'moveable'

- Whilst attention can be directed, this is often an effortful and difficult process

- It is hard to hold attention in one place! Often it wanders off, or gets dragged into focusing on something else

- Attention can 'play the body' – that is, what we pay attention to 'lights up' in our mind, and our bodies, and what we don't pay attention to goes out of our mind – just as a spotlight lights up what it shines on, and puts everything else in darkness

- Like a camera, attention can have a zoom-lens-like effect, enlarging and giving greater detail to what it focuses on. It can open, expand or narrow our consciousness, particularly when guided by strong emotion.

Just as in the case of other aspects of our minds, scientists have found that there are ways we can develop and strengthen our attention skills. They've also found that strengthening our attention 'muscles' can lead to a variety of benefits for our physical and mental health. For example, by training our attention we may be more able to notice what we're thinking or feeling (for example, loops in our minds) and we can, if needed, shift our attention to something else. Being able to direct our attention to something specific can help us to 'play a different tune in the body', one that is less stress-inducing than that related to threat-focused attention.

In this next section, we are going to explore one particular way of cultivating attention: through practising *mindfulness*.

Mindfulness – An anchor for your mind

We can develop our skills in mindfulness in a variety of ways, and there are many great books that explore a broad variety of these practices in more depth than we will be able to do here. In the remainder of this chapter we are going to explore a number of practices that are sometimes referred to as 'focused attention' mindfulness exercises. In these practices, we learn how to focus our attention on a very specific thing, such as our breathing, an image or a sound. We also learn to recognise when our attention moves away from this focus, and without judging ourselves for this, gently bring our attention back on focus. As these practices involve a specific foci for our attention (for example, our breath, or sounds around us), it can be useful to see these as *anchored* practices. In other words, we focus our attention and awareness on a particular thing (for example, the breath), and return to this when we notice that our minds wander.

We will explore some of these – and give you an opportunity to practise them – through the remainder of this chapter. Often when we start to practise mindfulness, it can be helpful to listen to an audio file to guide our practice. For each of the exercises below, you can find corresponding audio files on www.overcoming.co.uk. We've outlined a number of other tips that people often find helpful when practising mindfulness in Box 8.1 below.

Box 8.1: Some tips to help with practising mindfulness exercises

Tips – ways to practise mindfulness exercises

You will discover as you move through this book that there are lots of different types of practices designed to help you develop your skills in mindfulness, breathing, imagery and compassion. We will start most of these in a similar way – that is, by creating the conditions in which practice is most helpfully facilitated. In a way, this is similar to how sportsmen and women warm up before an event, stretching their muscles and getting ready before engaging in the actual event itself. For the purpose of the practice in this book, it can be helpful to get into the habit of first engaging in the following four steps:

Step 1 – If you can, find a place that isn't too loud, and in which you are unlikely to be disturbed during your practice

Step 2 – Find a comfortable place to sit

Step 3 – Adopt an 'upright' posture in which your feet are on the floor, roughly shoulder-width apart. Sometimes people resonate with the phrase 'sitting tall'

Step 4 – Either close your eyes, or select a natural point to focus your vision in front of you (e.g. on the floor, or the wall).

These are of course guides, and it is important for you to find a way to 'warm up' that is helpful to you.

Finally, it's also important to take your time with these exercises. We would advise that you take each one in turn, spending five to ten minutes on each one every day, to start with. After a period of time (for example, a week or so), you can move on to having a go at another practice.

When you are ready, have a go at the following exercise:

Mindful Exercise 1: Mindfulness of Breathing

To start with, find a place to sit in an upright, but comfortable position. If you feel able, close your eyes, or else pick a point to focus on in front of you. When you are ready, gently direct your attention towards your breathing. Begin to notice the sensation of breathing in and out. If it helps, try finding a point of focus to concentrate on. Some people find it helpful to focus on the area around the tip of their nose, noticing the sensation of air as it moves in and out. Others prefer to pick a point in the centre of the chest, noticing sensations as the chest expands on the in-breath, and contracts on the out-breath. Some like to follow the flow of the breath, from the point of entry to the body at the nose, through the nostrils, down into the throat and the lungs on the in-breath, and then out of the lungs, up through the throat and finally out of the nose on the out-breath. It may also be helpful to notice your belly rising and falling as you breathe in and out.

Try these different areas to focus your attention on and see what feels OK for you. The key thing is just to notice the experience of each, as there are no right or wrong ways of doing this. It may be that you feel your breath is a little shallow or ragged – don't worry if this is the case. It is more important that you start to become aware of the process and sensation of breathing itself.

Again, just notice the sensation of the in- and out-breath, tracking the process with each breath in and out as if you were just watching or observing this with curiosity. As you do this, there will be times when your attention is taken away from focusing on your breath. This may be because thoughts pop into your mind (maybe about what you're doing, e.g. 'This is boring' or 'I can't do this', or maybe thoughts about what you need to do later in the day). It might be that you get distracted by sounds around you, or some discomfort somewhere in your body. When you become aware that your attention has drifted, gently notice this and move your attention back to your breathing. Mindfulness is learning to observe how your mind is working in any one moment. A key thing to hold in mind here is that mindfulness does not have a specific 'result', such as holding your attention in one place. The exercises are simply to develop the skill of knowing where one's mind is at any moment. So the more your mind wanders and the more you notice, the more mindful you are! So there's no need to be judgemental when your mind does wander, just bring your attention back to your breathing until you notice your mind is distracted again.

Continue this process for five minutes or so, gently noticing your attention and sensation of breathing in and out. Remember, your breath can always be the anchor of your attention, something that you can always bring your mind back to, again and again. For now don't worry about having to change the frequency, pace or depth of your breathing, just pay attention to however your breath is.

Self-reflection: So, how did you find this exercise? What learning points can you take from this?

_____

_____

_____

Box 8.2: Some tips to help you with your mindfulness practice

Tips – steps to help with mindfulness practice

- Don't worry if your attention drifts away from your breathing – this happens to all of us when practising mindfulness. In fact we need this to happen so that we can develop awareness of the shifting of our attention focus

- It doesn't matter whether your attention drifts just once during this time, or a thousand times – the key thing is to do the following:
  » try your best to remember to notice when your attention has drifted away
  » when you've noticed that your mind has drifted from your breath, with kindness, gently try and bring your attention back to noticing your breath

- Mindfulness is not about clearing thoughts from our mind – it's learning to pay attention to what we're experiencing in the 'here and now' without judging, overanalysing or trying to push things out of our mind

- Don't worry about having to change the frequency, pace or depth of your breathing at the moment; just pay attention to however the breath is

- Try not to worry too much if you find this process difficult, or you feel yourself getting fed up or even bored – try your best to notice these feelings or thoughts as another understandable distraction and gently return your attention to your breathing

- It takes effort to practise and develop your skills in mindfulness – but this isn't an effortful 'forcing' or facilitated by self-critical dialogue such as 'You idiot, come on! You should be able to do this'. When we practise mindfulness, we try to do this in a non-judging, kind and caring way. We learn to be mindful (observing) of the struggles we experience during our practice of these exercises and gently return our attention to the present moment.

Let's try another exercise, this time using our body as the anchor for our attention.

Mindful Exercise 2: Body Scan

Find a comfortable place to sit or lie down. If you feel able to, close your eyes, or if you'd prefer, just pick a spot to focus your gaze upon. Allow your attention to begin to rest in the present moment – if it helps become aware of the sensation of breathing in and out, noticing the flow of the breath as it moves in and out of your body. To start, first, as best as you can, just try and focus upon the 'outline' of your body – maybe you can get a quick sense of the points of your body that connect with the chair you're sitting in, or with the floor you're lying on – almost as if you can get an outline of your posture and overall sense of body. Spend thirty seconds or so just becoming familiar with this.

Now we are slowly going to focus in a more systematic way on your body. To start with, try and pay attention to the area around your feet and ankles. Spend thirty seconds or so just noticing whatever sensations are present in this part of your body. You might be able to notice particular parts of your feet and ankles, or conversely, parts that are more difficult to notice. If you feel your attention being pulled away – by thoughts, sounds or sensations in other parts of your body – just become aware of this and without judging or being critical of this, gently bring your attention back to the sensations present in your feet and ankles.

Now slowly move your attention to your shins, calves and knee area. Again, notice the different sensations that are present as you begin to pay attention to this area of your body. Spend thirty seconds or so just paying attention to whatever sensations are present there. Now shift your attention to the area around your upper legs and bottom. See if you can pay attention to the sensations in this part of your body, and where possible, become aware when your attention is pulled away by other thoughts or sounds. If this happens gently and kindly bring your attention back to this area of your body. Spend thirty seconds or so just noticing the sensations that are present in this part of your body. See if you can resist the temptation to judge, fight or block the sensation, if it's an unpleasant one.

Now gently move your attention further up your body, to the area around your stomach and lower back. Notice any sensations that are present here, again for half a minute or so. After a comfortable period of time, slowly move your attention to your chest and upper back area. Notice the sensations that are present here for thirty seconds or so. Allow your attention to move to your arms and hands, allowing an awareness of the different sensations that arise in this part of your body. Keep noticing when your mind moves away from noticing sensations here. Remember, it is completely normal for your mind to wander and without judging yourself for this, try and gently move your attention back to noticing the sensation in your arms and hands.

Finally, slowly shift your attention to the area around your neck, face and head. Notice the sensations that are present in this part of your body. For thirty seconds or so just try and be aware of whatever sensations are present.

Self-reflection: What did you make of that exercise? What learning points can you take from it?

_____

_____

_____

So far we have focused on aspects of our bodies as an anchor for attention. Whilst some people find this relatively easy to do, for others, focusing on the body can actually feel quite uncomfortable and activate the threat system. So in this next exercise we will be anchoring attention on an external source – sounds.

Mindful Exercise 3: Mindfulness of Sound

Find a comfortable place to sit, again adopting an upright posture. For thirty seconds or so, just become aware of your body sitting in the chair, and for a moment or so, your breath as it moves in and out of your body. When you feel ready, see if you can slowly allow your attention to broaden away from your body. Start to become aware of the sounds that you can hear around you. To start with, try not to reach out to the sounds, but rather be receptive as they arise and disappear around you. Let them come to you – you are in this moment, just paying attention to the sound as it arises. Become aware of the direction they arise in, and their nature – what their character is, volume, tone, pitch or whether they are constant or intermittent. Try to notice when your mind has become distracted – this might be by thoughts or concerns that pop into your mind or emotional reactions to the sounds – and once aware, try, to the best of your ability, bringing your mind back to noticing the sounds around you again.

For sixty seconds or so, see if you can focus your attention more purposefully on one sound that you can hear around you. Really try to use this as an anchor for your attention. Notice with curiosity the nature and characteristics of this and return to this sound if your mind wanders. After a while try to pull back from focusing on this sound and see if you can split your attention and notice or become aware of all of the sounds you can hear around you, so that no sound is paid more attention to than others. Repeat this process, focusing on just one sound for a period, and then pulling the focus back to become aware of all sounds.

Self-reflection: What did you make of that exercise? What learning points can you take from this?

_____

_____

_____

Beyond the anchor – noticing the shifting landscape of our minds

So far in this chapter we've been focusing our practice in a more directed, anchored way – to the body, breath and sounds. These exercises are often a good place to start, and it can be helpful to take a few weeks to concentrate on them. As you gain experience and confidence in your practice, it can be helpful to broaden the lens of your practice. In this next exercise, we are going to step back from trying to focus our attention on a particular 'thing' (for example, sounds or your breathing) and pay attention instead to whatever passes through our attention without trying to direct the mind to anything.

The intention in this exercise is just to notice and observe your experience – to become aware of, and hold lightly in attention, whatever passes through our consciousness. So, no matter whether these experiences are positive, negative or neutral – whether they are emotions, thoughts, sounds or smells – we can learn to become more aware of them. Crucially, we will also learn that by labelling these – and allowing them to move in and out of awareness without holding onto them or pushing them away – we can become more at ease within our own mind. Let's try the next exercise:

Mindful Exercise 4 – Mindful Labelling

Sit in a comfortable but upright position. Spend a few moments orientating your mind – becoming aware of whatever is most prominent in your consciousness. This may be a physical sensation – a discomfort, pain or sense of relaxation; it may be thoughts, emotions or memories – positive, negative or neutral. When you become aware of any mental or physical experiences, allow yourself to notice this as an experience, without either pushing it away or becoming entangled in it.

Imagine that the sensations you experience are like watching leaves falling, one at a time, from a tree in autumn. So whether these 'leaves' are thoughts, feelings, sounds or physical sensations, try to observe them as they occur, without getting overly focused on one leaf but being open and aware when the next one falls. To help with this practice, you may also experiment with labelling (or naming) your experiences as they emerge into your awareness. By providing a link and descriptor to what we are experiencing and noticing, we can create a bit of distance between us and that experience, and thus avoid getting caught up or blindly tangled in it. So, for example, if you become aware that you are worrying about something you have to do at work tomorrow, you might try saying out loud, or in your head, the word 'thinking' or specifically 'worrying'. If you notice feeling anxious, sad or angry, you might give a broad description 'emotion', or label it in a more specific way (e.g. 'anxiety' or 'sad' or 'angry'). You can also do this if memories come to mind ('memory') or physical sensations (e.g. 'discomfort' or 'pain').

Notice, as best you can, how these experiences (and the labels you give them) can come and go, rise and fall, in your awareness – you do not have to judge, fight, attach or push away from them. Rather, they are just moments of connection with mental and physical sensations. We can remain open in our awareness and curious, noticing these experiences as they come and go, change or stay the same.

Continue for five minutes or so to notice your experiences as they come and go in your mind, labelling them when you can.

Self-reflection: How did you find this exercise? Was it easier or harder than the focused attention exercises? How did it feel to try and label your experiences as they emerged into consciousness?

_____

_____

_____

_____

Common difficulties

Throughout this book, we will be asking you to try out practices like the ones in this chapter. Whilst our experience is that some people find these types of practices relatively straightforward and easy to take to, many others (in fact, most people – including ourselves!) find them difficult for a variety of reasons. We've outlined a list of some of the most common difficulties in Box 8.3 below. You might not experience all of these as, of course, everyone is different; however, it is likely that you will experience at least one of these at some stage during your practice. For each difficulty, we've included some hints and tips that we personally, and many of our clients, have found helpful.

Box 8.3: Common difficulties and helpful hints when practising mindfulness

Common difficulty	Helpful hints
I don't think I'm doing it right – when I practise, I keep getting distracted and forget what I'm supposed to be doing.	Great! No, seriously, this is OK. The key thing to remember is that *you will get distracted* – that your mind *will* wander off to all sorts of random things (and sometimes not so random things – such as things that stimulate or occupy your threat system). If you can, try to remember that when your mind wanders this is a cue for a moment of mindfulness in itself (i.e. to notice that your mind has wandered from what you were focusing on) and an opportunity for you to return to your original focus.
I've tried practising your exercises a few times and nothing has changed – I still feel lousy. I don't think things will change if I practise more.	Although in the end some people don't take to mindfulness, try your best to stick with it, and your practice, as the benefits can be slow to realise. Although it is understandable to want this to 'work', try to step back from being too 'goal' orientated and focused on 'it working' or you getting/ feeling 'better'. Instead, try to focus on the reasons

why you are spending time practising mindfulness and your motivation behind this – to help create the conditions of compassion for your struggles.

Remember, the exercise and musical instrument analogies. Would you expect to get fit, or be able to play the guitar, after just a few sessions in the gym, or lessons with a music teacher? Like any skill, with practice we are more likely to become skilled at noticing paying attention in a moment-to-moment way.

When I practise mindfulness it makes me feel tired and sometimes I fall asleep!	This happens to almost everyone who has practised mindfulness – including both of us! Try not to beat yourself up if this happens. If you feel too sleepy, try moving around a little or keeping your eyes open whilst you practise. If you find yourself falling asleep a lot, this could be a sign that your mind and body need sleep rather than mindfulness in that moment.
I feel I should be able to 'clear' my mind or not think of anything when I practise mindfulness.	Whilst this is a tempting thought – and a common belief about meditation – clearing the mind, or not having any thoughts, is not the purpose of mindfulness. Instead, try to remember that mindfulness is more about noticing one's thoughts, and, as best as you can, try and bring your attention back to a particular focus (e.g. your breath or body; sounds; an image).
When I practise mindfulness, I sometimes experience unpleasant feelings or sensations (for example, when focusing on my breathing, or certain parts of my body during a body scan).	It can be helpful to know that this is a common experience and so try not to worry too much if this is the case. Sometimes it is helpful to stop your practice if the feeling is too unpleasant. However, maybe you can see if, with a little more time, the feeling begins to decrease naturally. In Compassionate Mind Training (CMT) we would understand this unpleasant experience in terms

	of threat system activation. Later on in the book we will teach you ways to regulate this using your compassionate mind.
Although I understand that mindfulness can be helpful, it seems like too much effort and hard work, and will take too long for me to notice any positive difference.	We know where you're coming from! This is something we've both experienced when practising mindfulness (but also in other areas of life – such as exercise!). Try to recall your intention and motivation for reading this book – the reasons for committing to this. Remember your drive for things to be different in life, combined with your wisdom that almost always change can take time and effort. But change is possible.

Practising mindfulness in everyday life

The above exercises are often most helpful when practised in a protected way by creating a space and time that is quiet and uninterrupted, often away from the hecticness of daily life. Whilst practising these exercises over time can help us to become more observant and aware of our experiences during everyday life, we can also practise mindfulness whilst going about our daily lives. You can try this yourself. Think about an everyday activity – this could be doing the washing up, taking a shower, or making (and of course drinking!) a cup of coffee. How can you engage in this activity *mindfully* – that is, doing this whilst remaining aware of your experience and observing your sensations as they occur in the present moment? If you can, decide upon an activity that you would naturally do in a day – maybe one that you would be doing shortly after reading this chapter – and set your intention to do this in a mindful way. Let's take the example of making a cup of tea or coffee. You might start by being mindfully aware of the physical sensation of picking up a cup, opening the cupboard and putting a tea bag/some coffee in the cup. Next, you might pay attention to the sound of the water as you fill the kettle, and then the noise of water beginning to boil. Notice sounds as you slowly pour the water into the cup, and the smell of tea or coffee that is present. Finally, notice the taste, temperature and smells as you take sips of the liquid.

Self-reflection: What was this like? How did you find engaging in this everyday activity in a mindful way? Did you notice anything different to your normal experience of this activity?

_____

_____

_____

We can practise this type of informal mindfulness in many ways throughout our daily life. The key intention is to bring our attention to this moment – observing our experience, as we are experiencing it. A way of doing this – even if it's just for a minute or two – is to ground this in our body movement and, in particular, walking. Let's try this by following the next exercise.

Mindful Exercise 5: Mindful Walking

To try mindful walking, the first thing you need to do is just that – walk! If you can, find a place where you have enough space to take at least ten steps before having to turn around. As you begin to walk around, notice the physical sensations that are present in your body. Gently become aware of what it feels like, physically, to be walking around the space that you're in. See if you can slow down your walking, and pay as much attention as you can to what this feels like in your body. Maybe you can pay attention to the sensation at the point where your heel touches the floor, then the centre part of your foot, followed by your toes before noticing that your heel is lifting. Now notice that your next foot is touching down on the floor. Go through the same process of being aware of contact – heel, centre and toes.

Notice any thoughts that come into your head and notice when your mind becomes distracted. When this happens, gently bring your attention and awareness back to the physical movement of walking. As you continue this process, see if you can become aware of the subtle sensations in your feet, ankles, legs and body.

For the final practice of mindfulness in this chapter, we're going to focus on mindful eating. As you might guess from the title of this exercise, you need to do a little preparation and get some food ready for the exercise. It doesn't matter what food you have, although it may be easier to start with something you can hold with your fingers, such as a small piece of fruit, like a grape or an apple or a raisin. The exercise is really about how to bring mindful awareness to this process.

Mindful Exercise 6: Mindful Eating

Spend a few moments looking at the food in front of you. Pick up the food, and spend a few moments noticing its texture. Turn it around in your fingers, noticing its shape, contours and colour.

Really pay attention to this as much as you can. Squeeze it gently, and notice its size and weight. Slowly and mindfully, noticing the sensations in your arm, move the food up to your nose. Taking your time, notice its smell. Now taste the food – but again, slowly, paying attention to the texture, the different sensations of taste as you slowly chew the food, moving it around your mouth. When you have finished chewing, notice how it feels to swallow the food. Complete this practice by paying attention to the sensation in your mouth in the absence of the food.

Self-reflection: Take a few moments to reflect on engaging in everyday activities in a mindful way. How did you find this? Was this experience any different to how you would usually engage in these activities?

_____

_____

_____

Thinking about the coming days, which daily activities could you do in a mindful way? What would help you to remember to do this?

_____

_____

_____

Mindfulness log

Like learning any new skill, creating the intention and space to practise is often key. It can therefore be helpful to keep a log of your practice – and in particular, which type of practice you've engaged in, and for how long. This will enable you to track which mindfulness exercises you've been practising, as well as plan and schedule mindfulness practice into your week. Furthermore, monitoring your mindfulness practice will give you feedback on your progress, and a sense of achievement related to this. In Figure 8.1 overleaf, make a note of which practices you've been using, when (what time of day) you practised, and how long you practised for.

Self-reflection: Keep the log for a week or two and then have a look back. What can you learn from this about the type, frequency and length of your mindfulness practice?

_____

_____

_____

What can you learn from your log that might help you going forward with your mindfulness practice (e.g. time of day most helpful to practise, length of practice, intention to practise a variety of exercises)?

_____

_____

_____

Figure 8.1: Weekly Mindfulness Practice Record

Week beginning: _____	How long did I practise for?	What type of mindfulness exercise did I practise?	What did I notice during my practice? Any learning points?
Monday Time			
Tuesday Time			
Wednesday Time			
Thursday Time			
Friday Time			
Saturday Time			
Sunday Time			

Chapter summary

In this chapter we've spent time learning and practising mindfulness. We have covered some key areas:

What we have learnt together	My personal reflections on the chapter
1. We have learnt about the nature of our attention, and in particular, how it tends to bounce around a lot. 2. We have also learned that when our attention focuses on something, this thing 'lights' up in terms of our sensory awareness, whilst everything else goes into darkness (i.e. we don't notice what we don't focus our attention on). 3. That our attention can, with effort, be moved around to notice different things. 4. That developing mindfulness – the ability to pay attention in the present moment without judging – can be an important way of bringing changes to our difficulties. 5. That practising developing our attention and mindfulness skills can be difficult. In persevering with our attempts, we can try and be kind and accepting of ourselves, and the difficulties we might face.	

9 Cultivating the soothing system I – Body and breathing focus

'Breath is the finest gift of nature. Be grateful for this wonderful gift.'

– Amit Ray, Meditation: Insights and Inspiration

You may remember in Chapter 3 we outlined a model of how our emotion systems can be grouped by their function (see pages 21–44). One of these emotion systems is the *soothing system*. We discussed how this system is linked to a state of calm and stillness when we are not under threat, nor in a seeking or trying to achieve mind state. This system has sometimes been referred to as a 'rest and digest' system, and is linked to the endorphins and activation of the parasympathetic nervous system. With the emergence of mammals, and the importance of care, bonding and attachment throughout the life cycle, we think this system was recruited to play an important role in facilitating and responding to caring relationships.

We also learnt in Chapter 3 that when activated, the soothing system can play a powerful role in helping us to manage and deal with our own – and other people's – threat system (see pages 42–4). In this chapter we are going to explore how we can cultivate this system so that it can do just that. It is likely that practising mindfulness, as we did in the previous chapter, may help with this. As we discovered, mindfulness practice can help us to become aware of our threat mind, and take steps to bring ourselves to the here and now. In this sense it can help us to shift from a 'doing mode', to a 'being mode', enabling us to feel more grounded in the moment, which can, in turn, facilitate the process of dealing with the difficulties we face. We can further build on our mindfulness skills through a number of practices – including working with our body, our senses, and our breathing – to strengthen our soothing system. In this chapter we will explore some of these in a step-by-step way.

1. Body posture

Our bodies have a significant impact on how we feel. Try this brief experiment: fold your arms, holding them tightly towards the middle of your chest, and at the same time pull your shoulders in, crunching inwards in your stomach a little. Hold this posture for ten to fifteen seconds, and then let go. What did you notice? An increase in tension, stress and even a flutter of anxiety? Here's another brief experiment. Begin to pay attention to your breathing in a mindful, moment-by-moment way, just as we practised in the previous chapter (see pages 105–6). As you do this, allow your body to slouch and your head/chin to lower towards your chest. How does this feel inside you and how does it affect your awareness? People often report a feeling of heaviness or tiredness, or a slight dulling of their awareness.

What we can learn from these brief experiments is that our body posture can have an impact on our feelings, including stimulating our threat system. As one of our main goals is to help you find ways to bridge out of your threat system towards your soothing system, we will teach you how to embody and practise various physical states (such as postures and facial expressions) that may help you to feel more confident, grounded and open. Let's have a try with this.

Exercise 1: Bridging From Threat to Soothing – Helpful Body Posture

Spend a moment to find a comfortable place to sit, or if you would prefer, to stand. Take time to imagine how you might hold your body if you were feeling confident, grounded and open. Maybe you can think about the position of your feet. How do you feel if your feet are directly together, or spread out widely from each other? Maybe you can try somewhere in between – roughly shoulder-width apart – and notice a sense of groundedness or stability in your body doing this. Just focus on this for thirty seconds or so.

Now let's focus on your back and shoulders. See if you can sit up, nice and straight – almost as if there were a piece of string coming out of the top of your head and someone was very gently pulling you up, lengthening your back a little. Notice for thirty seconds how it feels to be sitting or standing like this. Now notice your shoulders and chest. See if you can allow your shoulders to feel relaxed, and your chest to be in an open and comfortable position. Again, just notice how that feels for thirty seconds.

To finish with, let's bring all this together. In a mindful way, notice and observe how it feels to hold this upright, grounded and open posture in your body, from your feet to your spine, shoulders and chest.

Self-reflection: What did you notice in the previous exercise? What was it like to adopt this posture?

_____

_____

_____

_____

2. Facial expression

Building on the body posture practice earlier, it can also be useful to consider how facial expressions may help us to bridge from the threat to the soothing system. Our face often shows the world what we are feeling inside, but there is evidence that changing our facial expression might even change our feelings. In fact, this was found by researchers when they asked students to watch a cartoon holding a chopstick in their mouths in a manner that triggered the same facial muscles as a smile versus holding the chopstick in a way that activated the frown muscles. Students reported the cartoon to be funnier in the first trial when the smile facial muscles were activated. Let's have a go at exercise 2: Friendly Facial Expression.

Exercise 2: Friendly Facial Expression

To test this out for yourself, spend a few moments mindfully paying attention to your breathing. After a while, gently bring a warm, friendly expression to your face – something that feels comfortable to your face. If it helps, briefly think of someone you're very fond of and allow your face to move into a warm expression whilst holding them in mind. Just notice for thirty seconds how it feels to hold this facial expression whilst breathing. Now allow your face to return to your neutral expression, and just be with your breathing rhythm for thirty seconds. See if you can return to your warm, friendly facial expression for another thirty seconds, again noticing how this feels in comparison.

Self-reflection: How did that feel for you? Did you notice any differences? Sometimes people find that although at first the friendly facial expression feels a little 'odd', it leaves them with a greater sense of calmness, lightness or warmth in comparison to their neutral facial expression.

---

3. Soothing rhythm breathing

The way we breathe can have a powerful effect on our body. People in a number of careers – musicians, singers, actors and sportsmen and women – are taught how to breathe in different ways to help them perform at an optimum level. This is because the way that we breathe has a significant impact upon parts of our nervous system, which in turn, impacts upon our feelings, behaviour and the way that we think. Most of the time breathing is an automatic, non-conscious process, controlled by a very old part of your brain (the brainstem). In your body, the major system that influences the rate of breathing is called the autonomic nervous system. The autonomic nervous system helps to regulate non-conscious bodily actions, such as digestion, respiration and heart rate, and it has two major branches. The *sympathetic nervous system* helps to guide the body's fight or flight response, and is linked to the threat system; these include increasing heart rate, blood pressure and pupil dilation (potentially to let in more light so that we can better detect a threat). The *parasympathetic nervous system* is often seen as complementary to the sympathetic nervous system. Although a simplification, one way that the parasympathetic nervous system has been conceptualised is in terms of its function to slow down or balance the influence of the sympathetic nervous system. This helps to lower heart rate and blood pressure, and to slow down the body to allow periods of rest and recuperation. Scientists have found that we can stimulate the parasympathetic system through bringing changes to our body. These include practising certain types of body posture and facial expression, and also practising certain types of breathing rhythms.

Learning to breathe

Given what we've just been learning about, and in particular, how breathing can be associated with stimulating the parasympathetic nervous system (and therefore, an aspect of the soothing system), we are keen to utilise this in Compassionate Mind Training (CMT). As breathing is something that we all do, we are going to explore and practise different types of breathing rhythms that might be helpful to you. In fact, there is now growing evidence that suggests learning certain types of breathing rhythms can change our physiology, which in turn can help with our feelings and thinking.

Working with the breath has been a core aspect of many ancient physical and spiritual practices such as meditation, yoga and Tai Chi. In CMT, one way we can begin to bring about a potentially more helpful and calming breath is to practise something that we refer to as Soothing Rhythm Breathing (SRB). We are going to start off with a general version of this practice, and then add to this as we move through the chapter. We will also blend this breathing practice with the body posture and facial expression exercises we introduced above. Exercise 3 focuses on creating a soothing rhythm breathing.

Exercise 3: Soothing Rhythm Breathing

Find a quiet place to sit. Take a moment to embody the grounded, confident and open posture you practised earlier in this chapter, with your feet on the floor at shoulder-width, spine upright and shoulders slightly back and chest open. Bring your head into an upright position and gently bring a friendly expression to your face. When you feel ready, bring your attention to your breathing in a mindful way. Notice the sensations that are present as you breathe in and out, and when your attention becomes distracted, bring it back to focus on your breath in a gentle and kind way.

Now, as you're gently holding your attention in the flow of your breath, see if you can find a soothing or calming rhythm breathing. Take some time to experiment with this – to explore what your breathing rhythm would be like if it had a soothing or calming quality to it. It may be that this rhythm is a slower and deeper rhythm that usual, but one that feels comfortable to your body. If you can, try to breathe in a smooth, even way. If you notice your attention moving away from your breath, or that you become distracted in any way, gently bring your attention back to your breath and tune back in to the calming or soothing quality of your breathing rhythm. Spend a good sixty seconds or so practising your soothing rhythm breathing.

See if you can imagine a sense of 'slowing down' in your body as you breathe out. It can also be helpful to notice your body feeling a little heavier as you breathe out, whilst your legs are supported by the chair and your feet grounded on the floor. Continue practising this breathing rhythm for another five minutes or so, mindfully noticing when your awareness is distracted from this focus, and gently bringing your attention back to rest in the flow of your soothing rhythm breathing.

Self-reflection: What was the experience of engaging your soothing rhythm breathing? What did you notice? Did you notice any differences between this breathing and the mindful breathing we practised in the previous chapter (see pages 105–6)?

_____

_____

_____

_____

If you can, try to practise this exercise for five to ten minutes each day. If that feels too long, one or two minutes is a good start. Over time, see if you're able to gradually lengthen the duration of this practice.

Box 9.1: Common difficulties whilst practising Soothing Rhythm Breathing

When starting to practise SRB, many people find this quite difficult. It is very common to find this difficult at first, so try not to worry if this is the case. In our experience, some of the most common difficulties people have when practising SRB are as follows:

Common difficulties	Helpful hints
I don't like trying to slow my breathing down – it feels uncomfortable and makes me feel anxious.	This is a common experience when practising this exercise. Sometimes it can be helpful to remember that you are not the only one who experiences this. There can be a lot of reasons why slowing our breathing can feel uncomfortable – but like many things that we feel uncomfortable or anxious about initially, with further practice and 'exposure' the anxious feelings can begin to reduce and we can find the exercise easier. For some people there may be health conditions that make this exercise difficult – if

	this is the case, just try to practise aspects of this exercise that feel OK and comfortable to you.
I don't feel any sense of soothing when practising this. Am I doing it wrong?	Many people tell us this. The word 'soothing' can be a little tricky, implying that the goal of the exercise is to make you feel soothed.
	Whilst some people do feel a sense of soothing, calmness or peacefulness (which is great!), really the purpose of this exercise is to help people experience a physiological and psychological slowing down – a sense of stillness or groundedness rather than the feeling of soothing.

Slowing things down further

After you've practised soothing rhythm breathing for a while, and are feeling more comfortable with the experience of slowing down or calming with your out-breath, you could take this one step further. There is recent growing evidence that slowing down our breathing rhythm to approximately five or six breaths per minute, combined with an even, deep breathing rhythm, can produce a particularly helpful physiological balance between your sympathetic and parasympathetic nervous systems. Whilst for some people practising soothing rhythm breathing leads to a slower breathing rhythm, for others it doesn't. Even for those who do manage to slow their breathing down, sometimes the breathing rhythm can be a little quicker than five to six breaths per minute. So we will now practise purposefully slowing our breathing rhythm down a little further. You might want to have a timer or watch handy so that you can time your breathing, if that helps.

Exercise 4: Learning to Slow Down – How to Slow Your Breathing

Find a quiet and comfortable place to sit. Take a moment to embody the grounded, upright, confident posture you have practised in the earlier exercises. If you feel comfortable, close your eyes. If not, rest your gaze directly ahead of yourself, with your head in an alert, upright position. Begin by bringing your attention to your breathing in a mindful way. Notice the sensations present as you breathe in and out. If you notice that your attention becomes distracted, and moves away from your breath, just observe this and gently try to bring your attention back to your breath, without judging or criticising yourself that this has happened.

Now, as you're gently holding your attention in the flow of your breath, gently try and bring a soothing or calming rhythm breathing to your body. This is likely to be a slower and deeper rhythm than usual, but one that feels comfortable and natural to your body. Try if you can to breathe in a smooth, even way. If you notice your attention moving away from your breath, or that you become distracted in any way, gently bring your attention back to your breath and tune back in to the calming or soothing quality of your breathing rhythm.

Now, see if you can slow your breathing down a little further. Sometimes it can be worth counting your breath to start with. For example, try breathing in to the count of five, with each count representing a second. Once you've got to five, hold for one second before breathing out for five seconds (again counting to five as you do so). Hold for the count of one, before breathing in again to the count of five.

Out-breath 1 – 2 – 3 – 4 – 5

Hold 1

In-breath 1 – 2 – 3 – 4 – 5

Hold 1

Out-breath 1 – 2 – 3 – 4 – 5

Hold 1

In-breath 1 – 2 – 3 – 4 – 5

Continue – roughly in this rhythm – for another two or three minutes, staying connected with your soothing rhythm breathing.

Self-reflection: What was the experience of further slowing down the breathing rhythm like?

_____

_____

_____

_____

Many people find it helpful to use their smartphones or computers to support them with these exercises. Sometimes they record their therapists taking them through one of the exercises, or download audio clips on their phones to listen to, especially to start with. You can also download apps onto your phone that can guide your practice and set the rate of breathing per minute (the Breathing Zone app is a good example of this). A helpful thing about these apps is that you can set your own pace of breathing and begin to slow this down only when you feel comfortable and ready to do so.

4. Language

Language, and the words we use to capture our experiences, can have a big impact upon our feelings. For many of us, certain words are naturally associated with irritation or frustration (for example, certain swear words), whereas other words – such as 'calm', 'peace' or 'warm' – are associated with positive emotions and feelings. We are going to explore how using certain phrases alongside our breathing practice may further help the process.

Exercise 5: Using Words with the Out-Breath

Spend a moment preparing your body for the practice – engaging in a relaxed, yet upright body posture and friendly facial expression (see pages 122–3). When you feel ready, slowly engage with your soothing rhythm breathing, and take your time just to experience the sense of slowing down in your body. As you feel comfortable with this, try saying to yourself (in your own mind) the words 'calm' or 'soothe' as you breathe out. Try practising saying the word really quickly, then say it much more slowly so that it stretches out almost as long as your slow out-breath. Practise this for thirty to sixty seconds, just noticing what it feels like. Once you've done this, quietly continue to rest your attention in your soothing rhythm breathing for a short while.

Now, experiment with a different set of words. So the next time you breathe out, say the words 'mind slowing down' inside your head, in a slow even way that matches the length of your out-breath. Try saying this on the out-breath for the next minute. Now, try saying 'body slowing down' every time you breathe out, again in a slow even way that matches your out-breath. You may feel that there is another word or phrase that you can use to help this process of slowing down with the out-breath.

Self-reflection: How did this feel? What was it like to use language alongside your soothing rhythm breathing? Did you find a word(s) that helped the experience of the practice?

_____

_____

_____

5. Voice tones

From our formative experiences in life (and even before we are born), the voice tone of key people in our life (typically our parents) has a significant impact on our physiology. Scientists have found that after being placed in a stressful situation, children who heard their mother's voice experienced an increase in their oxytocin levels – the neuropeptide we mentioned in Chapter 3 that is related to bonding, closeness and trust (see pages 32 and 43), and the reduction of the stress hormone cortisol, amongst other things. We're now going to use these insights, by integrating voice tone to our soothing rhythm breathing practice.

Exercise 6: Voice Tone

As we've done throughout this chapter, take a few moments to prepare for the practice by embodying your grounded posture and friendly facial expression (pages 122–3). When you feel ready, slowly bring your soothing or calming rhythm breathing to your body, and spend a minute or so allowing yourself to slow down a little. Similar to the last practice, bring to mind words that you can repeat on the out-breath that help you to either focus on slowing down (for example, 'mind slowing down' or 'body slowing down'), or connect with the feelings associated with the soothing system (for example, the words 'calm' or 'soothe'). Now, as you're doing this, imagine that your inner voice tone is full of warmth, care and kindness. If it helps, again imagine the voice tone you might use with someone you feel really fond of and/or caring towards, and use this as the tone to say these words on the out-breath. As ever, notice when your attention is distracted, mindfully bringing awareness back to your voice tone. Continue to practise this, your warm, kind and caring voice tone repeating a word or phrase every time you breathe out.

Self-reflection: What was it like to use a caring and warm voice tone in this practice? What impact did it have on your experience of your breathing rhythm, or on how you felt?

_____

_____

_____

6. Focus of attention

Some people who practise breathing find that an explicit focus on the inner experience of this is uncomfortable, anxiety provoking or distressing in some way. One way of helping with this is to keep the same, slower and deeper breathing rhythm, but focus one's attention outside of the body. This can be done by holding an object, such as a stone, a set of beads, a ball, or any other small object that has a soothing, comforting or calming texture to you. As you engage your breathing rhythm, hold the object in your hand, focusing on the texture and the feeling of this. You can also do this by using technology. We mentioned previously that mobile phone and computer apps can be helpful in learning how to pace your breathing (see pages 126–7). However, many of the people we see for therapy, and many psychologists and therapists that we've taught, have found that by focusing their attention on the app (often an image that changes shape or size to guide your breathing rhythm) helps to take attention away from the body, whilst the body (breath) still engages in a helpful rhythm.

Self-reflection: Were you able to find an object that had a grounding or soothing quality to it? If you used an app to focus your attention outside your body, what was that like? What effect did it have on your experience of soothing rhythm breathing?

_____

_____

_____

7. Smells

Similarly to sounds, certain smells can either elicit negative responses in us (think about the smell of out-of-date eggs!), or positive ones (the smell of jasmine, or freshly made coffee or baked bread). Using this idea, it can be helpful to spend some time trying out different smells, finding one has a soothing or calming quality for you. Different people find different smells helpful with this – lavender or rose oil, for example, or something completely different. Once you've found something, engage with your soothing rhythm breathing whilst gently focusing your attention on the smell you've selected. Continue with your breathing rhythm while noticing the smell for another two or three minutes.

Self-reflection: Were you able to find a smell that was soothing or calming in some way? How did it affect the experience of your soothing rhythm breathing practice?

_____

_____

_____

8. Sounds

Most of us have experienced directly how music can change our mood; our favourite songs can often leave us feeling happy, excited, sad or calm. Think about what sort of music leaves you feeling calm or peaceful. Similarly, certain sounds – for example, that of a river or the sea, the wind moving through the trees, or birds singing – can have a calming, grounding effect on us. When you've found a piece of music or a sound with a calming quality to it, see if you can have this on in the background whilst you're practising your soothing rhythm breathing.

Self-reflection: How did this leave you feeling? Was it helpful in your practice, or distracting? Maybe it would be helpful to practise with different background sounds to see if there is something that works better for you.

_____

_____

_____

Summary Exercise: Developing a soothing kitbag

We've explored a number of ways that we can stimulate the physiology of the soothing system. Sometimes people find it helpful to develop a 'soothing kitbag'; these may be a combination of exercises, sounds, images, smells or objects that help you to access your soothing system when you need to. It might help to start by making a list of what these might be for you, and then over time, bring them together somewhere (a box, bag or on your smartphone) where you can access them easily.

My soothing kitbag: things that help my soothing system

1. _____

2. _____

3. _____

4. _____

5. _____

6. _____

Putting your skills to work – soothing breathing

The skills and practices that we introduced in this chapter, and the previous chapter on mindfulness (see pages 101–19), have been shown to bring about positive changes to our minds and bodies. Beyond such immediate benefits to our wellbeing, these skills can help us to manage our threat system when it is activated. This is similar to regular physical exercise: not only does going to the gym regularly lead to positive physiological changes over time, but it also increases our fitness, which in turn allows us to do certain things more efficiently and effectively – for example, running to catch a bus, participating in a marathon to raise money for charity, or competing in a football match.

With this analogy in mind, it can be helpful to begin using soothing rhythmic breathing in 'real life' scenarios. This can help you develop the confidence and awareness of how using this exercise can have day-to-day applications. It may be helpful to try the following:

1. Begin by practising slow soothing breathing whilst you're with someone that

you feel comfortable with (for example, sitting on the sofa next to someone watching TV, but not talking).

2. Next, try and practise this whilst you are in a conversation with someone you feel safe and comfortable with. It can take a while to get used to learning to breathe more slowly whilst also engaging in conversation but keep on trying – this often gets easier.

3. Finally, see if you can engage in this type of breathing when your threat system is activated. Again, this might feel hard at first, but remember, if we can stimulate our soothing-affiliative system (and thus our parasympathetic nervous system), this can help us to regulate our threat emotions.

Chapter summary

There are many ways that we can influence our feelings and physiology. In this chapter we've explored how focusing on our senses and bringing changes to our body – through breathing, body postures and facial expressions – may help to stimulate aspects of the soothing system. Take your time and experiment with the different skills and practices we've introduced here. In time, you'll be able to form your own combination of the ones that work best for you.

What we have learnt together	My personal reflections on the chapter
1. We can use a variety of practices and skills to help bridge from threat system towards soothing system. These include mindfulness, body posture and particular types of breathing rhythms. 2. Practising a soothing rhythm breathing that is slower than our usual breathing pace can help to stimulate the soothing-affiliative system. 3. We can further cultivate the soothing system by 'adding' various sensory foci to our soothing rhythm breathing. These include certain smells, sounds and facial expressions. 4. Learning to use these skills can help us to tolerate and manage our threat system.	

10 Cultivating the soothing system II – Using imagery and memory

'Knowledge is limited. Imagination encircles the world.'

– *Albert Einstein*

In the previous chapter we looked at how to activate the soothing-affiliative system using our body, senses and breathing. Most of this focused on stimulating the underlying physiology of the soothing system, helping to create a sense of slowing, groundedness and calming. In this chapter we are going to continue to focus on developing the soothing-affiliative system, but this time we are going to do this through the use of imagery and memory. In particular, we're going to explore ways of activating this system in the context of affiliative (caring) relationships.

What is imagery?

There are a number of different definitions of what imagery is. From a psychological point of view it is sensory information experienced in the mind that does not have a direct environmental trigger or input. Mostly, when we consider imagery, we think of visual imagery, which is the ability to create or experience visual pictures in our minds. However, we can experience the types of imagery described below through the whole range of our senses:

*   Visual imagery – this involves generating visual images in our minds, such as imagining the shape and colour of a tree, or the visual characteristics of a person

*   Auditory (sound) imagery – this involves imagining sounds, such as the sound of the waves against the shore, or a wood pigeon calling

*   Olfactory (smell) imagery – this involves bringing to mind certain smells, such as freshly cut grass

*   Tactile (touch) imagery – this involves imagining certain tactile sensations, such as the feel of grass or sand under our feet, or the warmth of the sun against our skin

- Taste imagery – here, images focus around our sense of taste; for example, imagining the taste of coffee, or our favourite food.

Why is imagery helpful for stimulating the soothing system?

Although imagery, by its very nature, is not 'real' in the same way that we experience things around us in the world, it can still result in the same type of experiences in our body as if it were real. One way that we can understand this is through Figure 10.1 below, which we will talk you through.

Figure 10.1: How the brain responds to internal triggers in the same way as external triggers

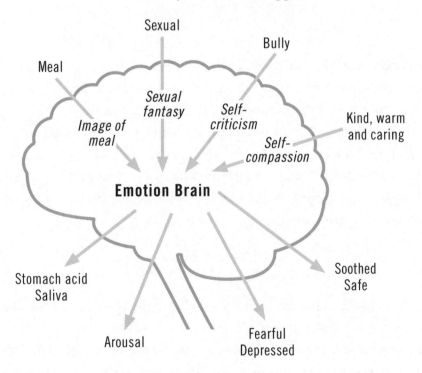

Adapted from Gilbert, *The Compassionate Mind* (2009), reprinted with permission from Constable & Robinson Ltd.

Example 1

The first example to think of is food. Have a think for a moment about what your favourite food is, and consider, if you hadn't eaten all day, what might happen in your body upon seeing and smelling it in front of you? Maybe a little rumbling in your stomach or saliva in your mouth? This happens because the sight and smell of the food stimulates a part of your brain (the pituitary), which, in turn causes a cascade of physiological responses that lead to your body getting ready to digest the food.

Now, just imagine your favourite food in your head – really pay close attention to this, imagining its smell, taste and texture. What do you notice if you really focus on this image? Maybe saliva in your mouth, or your stomach rumbling a little? So although there is no real food, or no actual lemon, the image of it stimulates the same parts of our brain as the real thing does, and therefore leads to the same physiological response in the body.

Example 2

Let's take a second example. Think about what happens when you are with your partner or someone that you find very sexually attractive and things are becoming a little steamy! What happens in your body? Well, without getting too graphic, this stimulates part of your brain, which in turn stimulates parts of your body, leading to you feeling sexually aroused. However, do you need a real person for this to happen? Well, no – you can just close your eyes and imagine or fantasise about someone you find attractive, and this imagery will lead to the same thing – sexual arousal in your body. This is, again, because imagining someone sexy stimulates the same parts of the brain as the real thing.

Example 3

Think about what would happen if you were being bullied by your boss and colleagues at work over a period of many months. How might that affect you or leave you feeling? Maybe a little low in mood, stressed, anxious or angry? We know that this may be the case because the experience of threat and hostility from others triggers our threat systems and the physiological processes (e.g. stress hormones) linked to it, and that over time, this can lead people to feel stressed and low in mood. Of course we don't need a 'real' experience like this to end up feeling stressed and low. We can remember hostile 'voices', or even criticise and bully ourselves, and end up feeling exactly the same. Researchers have found that self-criticism and self-directed hostility may be vulnerability factors for depression and anxiety, or maintain mental health distress. And even though we can potentially escape from the hostility and criticism of bosses, colleagues and others by taking time off and surrounding ourselves with friendly people, when it comes to our inner critic we hardly have a break and instead can feel trapped. To make matters worse, this inner critic knows our vulnerabilities and uses them against us. We will come back to look at self-criticism in more detail in Chapter 23.

Example 4

It can be helpful to think about how the effect of imagery might apply to our soothing-affiliative system and, more broadly, compassion. Think about how it feels if you are surrounded by friends and family who are kind, caring and compassionate to you. How might that leave you feeling? Maybe with a sense of safety, connectedness or an inner experience of calm? We know this can happen because such interactions of care and support stimulate our soothing-affiliative system, triggering neurophysiological responses that give rise to the feeling of soothing and safety. Of course it's very nice when we have supportive friends and family around to help us feel safe. But, in their absence, we can generate the same feelings by imagining kind and caring others, or even developing our own internal voice of compassion – in other words, cultivating our self-compassion.

Summing up

Hopefully the above examples, including Figure 10.1, are helpful in highlighting some important reflection points about imagery:

- Although real events in the world around us and images or fantasies in our mind are different, they can stimulate the same parts of our brain and leave us with the same felt experience

- On one level our brains do not discriminate well between externally derived signals (real events in the world) and internally derived signals (mental images)

- Deliberately practising certain types of images (for example, those linked to the soothing-affiliative system) may be an important step in helping to build the soothing-affiliative system and compassion.

Recent scientific findings have found that imagery has a bigger impact on our emotions than words alone, and that certain types of soothing imagery practices were linked to lower levels of stress hormones. This suggests that imagery could be a powerful tool when working with difficult emotions linked to our threat system. The next steps in this chapter involve imagery practices that can stimulate the soothing-affiliative system.

Expectations about imagery

Sometimes when we talk of imagery, and of creating images, people can have expectations of what we mean, and of what they should be trying to create. For example, some people feel that they should have HDTV, 3D visual images, which are clear and stable. For most people (including us), imagery is most often fleeting, transient and short-lived. Here are some examples that might help to understand what we mean by imagery. Consider the following questions:

What does a tree look like?

What does a car look like?

What does your kitchen table look like?

Whatever popped into your mind in trying to answer these three questions – this is imagery. Nothing more, nothing less. Now, that isn't to say imagery is easy! We are simply helping you understand what we are hoping to do in the following imagery exercises.

Imagery practice – Developing the soothing system

As we progress through this book, you will see that imagery forms an integral part of the change process, used to help you develop different skills and abilities. In the following section we are going to use imagery exercises to work on cultivating and building the soothing system.

Exercise 1: Soothing Colour Imagery

Sit in an upright but comfortable position, adopting a grounded and confident body posture. Engage in your soothing rhythm breathing (see pages 126–31) for a minute or so, allowing your body to slow down by finding a calming rate of breathing. When you're ready, imagine a colour that you find calming, soothing or peaceful. Take your time with this, mindfully observing what colour, or colours, come to mind. Try not to worry if you find this difficult – if it helps, bring your awareness back to your soothing breathing and after a while, try to bring a soothing colour to mind.

When you are ready, imagine your soothing colour in front of you. Maybe you could imagine it taking the form of light or mist. After a moment, imagine this soothing light or mist is moving towards you, slowly surrounding and supporting you. Notice how having this soothing or calming colour surrounding and supporting you leaves you feeling inside. If you can, imagine this colour has an awareness – it wants to support you, help you feel soothed and calm. Focus on this for sixty seconds or so.

Create a friendly or warm facial expression. You might want to imagine that this colour is entering your body through the area around your heart, and moving through your body, soothing and calming you. Continue mindfully paying attention to this image for another two or three minutes, noticing the sensations that are present as you do.

Self-reflection: How did you find this exercise? If you were able to imagine a colour, maybe you could describe it below. How did this leave you feeling?

_____

_____

_____

What was it like to imagine that the colour had a caring and supportive intention towards you?

_____

_____

Common difficulties with soothing colour exercise

Some people find imagining a soothing colour a little difficult at first. In Box 10.1 below we have outlined a number of common difficulties that people we worked with have shared, with some hints and tips on what might help with each.

Box 10.1: Common difficulties and helpful hints for soothing colour

Common difficulties	Helpful hints
I found it difficult to bring any images to my mind.	This is probably the most commonly reported difficulty. Consider what made this difficult – for example, whether your mind was getting distracted, or you became critical with yourself for not being able to 'do' the practice. If this is the case, try your best to use your mindfulness skills to gently refocus your mind.
I had an image for a while, but it wasn't very clear and then I lost it.	It can be really frustrating when this happens. It might be helpful to engage your mindfulness skills (see pages 101–19) to notice this as an experience, trying not to get caught up with frustration and instead gently return to your intention to pay attention to the image of your soothing colour.
I found it hard to think of a colour that is soothing.	It can be helpful to start by paying attention to colours around you – in your home, office or the area that you live in – noticing whether any leave you feeling calm in some way. If you have access to a computer, type into Google 'calming colours' or 'soothing colours' and see what comes up. You can then use this to guide your practice.

Creating a Calm, Peaceful and Safe Place

In this next exercise we are going to try and create an image of a place that will help you to connect with the soothing-affiliative system and related feelings, such as safety, calmness, contentment, peacefulness and so forth. This place could be somewhere that you've been to, somewhere you've seen on TV or the internet, or somewhere completely made up or fantasy based. The key thing is for this place to allow you the feelings associated with the soothing-affiliative system.

Here are a few examples that have previously been developed:

Celina's safe place was a golden beach, with beautiful soft, warm sand and crystal-blue water. She imagined the warm sunlight against her skin, the soft sound of the water lapping against the shore, and the smell of pine needles from the forest behind the beach.

Carter's image was of his garden. He was able to bring to mind the vibrant colourful flowers in summertime and the sound of birds in the trees, as well as the soft, calming sound of the water pond. He could also imagine the wind against his skin.

Jade created a fantasy image. This was of a huge forest, with a beautiful, grassy clearing, with an old, tall but soft tree in the middle. She imagined the tree had arms and gently held her with these warm, comforting arms.

Your safe place may be similar or very different to these – the main thing is to develop an image with the intention that is has the quality of safety, calmness, peacefulness or tranquillity. Try not to worry about getting this right or wrong, just try and think about what sort of place this would be.

Exercise 2: Creating an Image of My Safe Place

Find somewhere comfortable to sit where you will not be disturbed. Take a few moments to adopt your grounded, upright, confident body posture. Engage in your soothing rhythm breathing (see pages 126–31), allowing your breathing and body to slow down a little.

When you feel ready, spend some time bringing to mind an image of a place that you feel is safe, soothing or calming in some way. This may be somewhere you have been before or somewhere completely 'made up'. Try not to get frustrated or worried if no image comes to mind for a while, or if you find that several different images come to mind. Mindfully try and stay with the intention to allow an image to come to mind that feels safe, calming or soothing in some way.

When an image has come to mind, spend a few moments being with it. To start with, mindfully pay attention to what you can see in this image. This might be colours, shapes, or objects. Spend thirty seconds doing this. Next, notice if there are any sounds that are present in this image or your safe place. If there are, gently pay attention to these, noticing the different qualities they may have, how they leave you feeling. Spend thirty seconds or so doing this. Now, notice whether there are any soothing or comforting smells that are present here in your image. If there are, again, spend thirty seconds paying attention to this. Next, notice any physical sensations you can feel or things you come into physical contact with or touch, such as the warmth of the sun against your skin or the feel of the grass, or sand beneath your feet. Focus on this for thirty seconds. Maybe you can consider whether you are in your safe place on your own, or whether someone or something else (like an animal), is there with you.

As this is your own safe place, imagine that it has an awareness of you. It welcomes you there, and is happy to see you; it wants you to feel safe and calm. Notice how it feels to know that this place wants you to feel supported, safe and at ease. Spend a minute or so just focusing on this.

Given that this is a place in which you can feel at ease, calm and safe, it may be useful to consider what you would like to do whilst being here. Maybe you wish to remain still, content with just 'being' in the moment, in this place. Or you might like to explore the place in a more active way, or moving around in this place, walking, swimming or playing a game. It is your own unique safe place, you can use it in a way that helps you to feel at ease, as well as engaged and interested, with the freedom to explore.

Self-reflection: How did you get on with this exercise? What was it like to create an image of a place where you could feel safe, calm and peaceful?

_____

_____

_____

Make a few notes on the image you generated. What could you see? What could you smell or hear? What tactile sensations did you notice?

_____

_____

_____

What was it like to imagine being welcomed and supported by your safe place?

_____

_____

_____

Difficulties with safe place imagery

Whilst many people find this imagery practice quite powerful, like the other exercises we've explored in this workbook, some common difficulties are often reported. Take a look at Box 10.2 below, which outlines some of these with some ideas about what might be helpful.

Box 10.2: Common difficulties and helpful hints for safe place imagery

Common difficulties	Helpful hints
I couldn't think of any image to bring to mind.	This is one of the most common difficulties with this exercise. Try not to get disheartened. There are a number of things that could help: • It can be hard trying new things for the first time – but like most things, this is likely to get easier over time

	• Spend some time before you practise to remember any places you've been to that have the qualities of calmness, soothing or safety • Have a look at images in magazines or the internet for inspiration • The place does not have to exist in reality, or be one you have visited. It can be a place of fantasy, somewhere you've completely made up, or a mixture of different places you've been to.
Several different images came to mind, and I struggled to focus on just one of them.	Although it might seem that having a lot of possibilities for your image would be a good thing, in practice it can often make it harder. See if you can use your mindfulness skills (see pages 101–19) to notice your mind jumping to these different images, and see, with the help of your soothing rhythm breathing, whether you can settle your mind to one of the images. Remember, you may start with one image, but change it or move to another over time. If it helps, you can try and mix your images together. In the end, it's your safe place and you can make it anything you'd like it to be.
I couldn't visualise anything in my place.	Remember, visual imagery is only one component of imagery – see if it is easier to imagine smells, sounds or tactile sensations. Sometimes people find it helpful to have an actual picture of a calm or soothing place as a prompt for this imagery exercise.

Box 10.3: Some tips to help with safe place imagery

Tips – for safe place imagery

- The word 'safe' can trigger bad memories for some people. If this is the case for you, try words like 'comforting', 'peaceful' or 'calming place' instead.

- If you struggle to feel safe in your place, it could be helpful to ask yourself: 'What do I need for this place to feel safe?' or 'What quality do I need to make this safe?'

- Remind yourself of how our 'tricky brains' work and that the purpose of developing compassion is to regulate the threat system.

Boosting the signal

Whilst imagery can be a powerful tool for stimulating our physiology and feelings, we can also experiment with ways to trigger our senses that may boost or amplify the feelings associated with this imagery practice. Similar to Chapter 9 (see also pages 130–1), we've outlined a few ideas below which can be used alongside the safe place imagery exercise. See how it feels to try some of these out for yourself.

- Vision – some people find it very helpful to start this exercise by being able to first look at, and use, a real image of a place that they can then build their image from. To do this, you may want to look through some old photos from trips or holidays you've been on, or take a photo of an actual place you visit. For inspiration, you might want to type in to Google 'safe place' or 'calming place' and see what images come up, or, if you know the type of place you are looking for, you may search for that (e.g. beautiful beach or garden). Once you find one they like, have this to look at whilst doing the imagery exercise.

- Sounds – sometimes people find it helpful to play certain music in the background whilst engaging in the safe place imagery practice. Maybe you can experiment with different types of sounds or music that can help you to connect with your safe place – for example, the sounds of a flowing stream, or of a forest, or maybe some classical music.

- Smells – many of us realise that smells have a powerful impact on the way we feel. In a negative way, certain smells (rotten eggs, methane gas!) provoke a strong negative aversive feeling in us. Other smells – for example, freshly cut grass or lavender – can leave us with a sense of calm and contentment. Do any smells come to mind that help you to feel calm? It might be worth taking a trip to an essential oils shop and trying out different smells to find one that generates a soothing response in you.

- Touch – our tactile sense, what we can touch and feel, can help to stimulate our soothing-affiliative system. Sometimes holding an object that helps us to feel grounded (for example, holding a stone) or something that reminds us of feelings of care, soothing or calmness (e.g. a picture of our children or loved ones) can generate these very feelings. Some people find it helpful to have an object that has a soft, silky or soothing touch to it – for example, a velvety or fluffy piece of material. Other people generate this inner calm by using their own touch, stroking one hand with the other, or gently resting both hands at the centre of the chest, or just over their heart area.

Self-reflection: What was it like to 'boost the signal' of your safe place imagery by using some of the suggestions above? Did you notice any differences?

_____

_____

_____

Developing the soothing–affiliative system – using memory

So far in this chapter we have used imagery to stimulate the soothing-affiliative system. Another way we can help you to stimulate and cultivate this system is from memory. Some of you may have used your memory when you were practising the image of the safe place. You may have brought to mind the memory of an actual place that you find calming and peaceful and used that to build your imagery around. We are going to take a similar approach here and see if we can use memory to recall a time when we experienced receiving care, support, and kindness from another person, which resulted in us feeling safe, calm and content. The key thing during this next practice is to try to build it around a memory of a time when you were not struggling too much or were overly distressed, as this is likely to stimulate your threat system and change the nature and function of the exercise.

Exercise 3: Memory of Feeling Cared For

Find somewhere comfortable to sit where you will not be disturbed. Engage in your soothing rhythm breathing (see pages 126–31), allowing your breathing and body to slow down a little. If you can, bring a friendly expression to your face. Spend sixty seconds or so doing this.

When you feel ready, try to bring to mind a memory of a time when you felt calm, content or connected – for example, when somebody was being warm, kind or caring towards you. This person might be somebody you care for, and/or who cares for you very much. Or it could be someone you don't know well, or even a stranger. The key thing is that it is a memory of a time when you were left feeling calm, safe and connected following the actions of another person. Spend thirty to sixty seconds allowing your mind to connect with this memory.

We are now going to spend some time paying attention to specific aspects of this memory. To start with, see if you can recall where you were: notice the environment around you, and where the other person was in relation to you (for example, in front of you or by your side). Now take a moment to pay attention to this other person. Maybe you can notice their facial expression, body posture or voice tone that somehow conveyed their caring and supportive intentions towards you. Don't worry if you can't specifically remember these – just imagine what they might have been like instead. Given the qualities of this person and what they were doing for you, see if you can remember what it felt like to receive this kindness and care from them. Pay attention to any feelings of safety, contentment or connection. Spend sixty seconds or so paying attention to the feelings emerging from the way that someone else treated you. When you feel ready, slowly bring your attention back to your soothing rhythm breathing and gradually bring this exercise to a close.

Self-reflection: So, how did you get on with that exercise? How did it feel to bring back to mind this memory of receiving care and support?

Whilst many find this exercise very powerful, sometimes it can trigger feelings of *loss* – feelings of sadness or anger towards the person who was kind to us (maybe through a breakdown of the relationship, or even death), or grief related to not having those types of experiences in life itself. Although unpleasant, we can see these feelings as an understandable response to being reminded of people who are no longer in our lives, or an indication of what we naturally need (i.e. human closeness and connection). It can also be helpful to recognise them as linked to activation of the threat system, and therefore an opportunity to engage with some of the skills you've been developing in recent chapters to help manage these feelings (e.g. mindfulness, soothing breathing or safe place imagery). If it feels OK to practise the memory exercise again, it might be helpful to bring a different memory to mind and see how that feels in comparison.

Chapter summary

Following on from Chapter 9, here we've continued to focus on ways of developing and stimulating the soothing system.

What we have learnt together	My personal reflections on the chapter
1. That imagery can be a powerful tool in stimulating our feelings and physiology. 2. How practising imagery – soothing colour and safe place – can stimulate our soothing system and leave us feeling calm and safe. 3. That imagery can involve different senses – vision, sound, smell and tactile experiences.	

11 Building the drive system

'Strength does not come from physical capacity; it comes from indomitable will.'

– Mahatma Gandhi

Although we have prioritised the cultivation of the soothing-affiliative system so far in this section of the book, we are also interested in how we can develop and have access to a healthy drive system. If you recall from Chapter 3, the drive system plays an important role in motivating the pursuit and acquisition of resources – for example, food, shelter and sexual opportunities. It is associated with wanting, pursuing, seeking and consuming. These desires, behaviours and motives are likely to have increased our ancestors' chances of survival, and as a consequence, the likelihood of them passing on their genes through reproduction.

The drive system is linked to certain types of positive emotions that are quite different to those linked to the soothing-affiliative system (for example, contentment and calmness), discussed in previous chapters. These emotions include excitement and joy, and the energised feelings we experience when we succeed or win or get something we want. Such feelings also operate as positive reinforcers, meaning that they make us more likely to want to engage again in the same behaviours that led to these feelings. The drive system, and the emotions we experience when this is activated, is associated with a chemical called dopamine that, amongst other things, is linked to a sense of energy, pleasure and reward. It is also linked to the sympathetic nervous system, which gets the body up and ready for action.

As we discussed in Chapter 3 (see page 37), the experience of this system can be a little tricky. Western culture places a great emphasis on drive, which can bring both pleasure and distress, and sometimes more distress than pleasure. Our school systems and society commonly place great importance on being 'the best' and succeeding, and often value this as the hallmark of a living a 'good', fulfilling life. Our political and social systems often focus on competition, success, acquisition of resources and money, whilst media and advertising companies promote images of what we should look like (e.g. thin, attractive) and what material goods we should have (e.g. clothing, bags, jewellery or cars), with subtle (or not so subtle) messages that unless we have these things we will be unhappy. So there is a lot of emphasis in our society on the drive system – both on its related emotions (e.g. pleasure and excitement), and the motives underpinning it (pursuing, competing and the acquisition and consumption of things). As we discussed in Chapter 3, the motive to compete and achieve can, for some of us, be closely linked to the threat system. In other words, we can desperately strive to be successful to avoid and manage feelings of inferiority and inadequacy. For other people, particularly individuals who experience considerable anxiety and low mood, the drive system may become blocked, or underactive. If this is the case, it can be difficult to pursue, engage in, and take pleasure from activities and things that are important and helpful in our lives (for example, one's career, or socialising with friends).

Whilst it is important to be aware of the potential unhelpful interactions between the threat and drive systems, we do not wish to demonise the drive system, or the emotions linked to it. In fact in this chapter we are going to think about how we can learn to create a healthy, sustainable and balanced drive system. As we'll come to see, one way that we can do this is by activating the drive system from a position of groundedness and stability. We will therefore use the skills we developed in previous chapters linked to the soothing-affiliative system.

The drive system has some important implications for developing our compassionate minds. Compassion, as a motive driving behaviour, is not exclusively related to the soothing system; rather, it operates as the fulcrum of the three systems and is linked to all three (the threat, drive and soothing systems). Whilst the soothing system is linked to the caring motivation of compassion, which is needed to help us engage with distress and suffering (the threat system), we ultimately need the energy, desire and reward-seeking of the drive system to seek to engage with this distress, and actively try to alleviate suffering, or prevent it from returning. Moreover, compassion extends beyond suffering, and its alleviation. It carries a motivation for all sentient beings (including humans) to experience happiness, find meaning and purpose, and flourish. In this way, the drive system, with its energising and motivating impact, urging us to seek things that are meaningful and fulfilling, has an important role to play in developing our compassionate minds. We will explore all of this in detail in this chapter. Before we get started, though, you may find it helpful to have a look at the hints and tips in Box 11.1 below.

Box 11.1: Tips to help with creating a healthy drive system

Tips – creating a healthy drive system

- As you practise the exercises in this chapter, try to hold in mind what motive you are trying to access the drive system from. In particular, try to be aware if a competitive motive shows up, or if you become aware of 'threat-system activation', where you may experience a sense of striving to 'get it right', or a fear of not doing a good job. If this is the case, see if you can connect with your sense of care and commitment to yourself, being as encouraging and supportive to yourself as possible.
- In terms of the three-system model (see page 22), it can be helpful to try and engage in these exercises from a counter-clockwise, rather than clockwise position. So, rather than doing the drive system exercises from the threat system (clockwise into the drive), try instead to connect with the grounding and stability aspect of the soothing system first, before engaging in the practice.
- It is also worth holding in mind that the following exercises are likely to blend both drive and soothing systems, rather than the drive system alone. The neurophysiological processes involved in these experiences are complex, and the three-system model is only a heuristic for simplifying these processes in an understandable way.

Developing the drive system

There are many different ways of cultivating the drive system. Here, we will look at two of these. We will start by focusing on how we can engage and guide our drive system in a particular way. We are then going to work on how we can use our attention to ensure we actively engage in opportunities to connect with the positive emotions linked to this system.

Box 11.2: Tips to help with compassion–based goals, values and motives

Tips – for compassion–based goals, values and motives

It can be helpful to bring to mind examples of compassionate goals, values or motives to base the following exercises on. These may include motives to:

- Help other people
- Be a good role model
- Experience the joy of being with other people, and sharing things with them
- Teach or share your knowledge with someone else who is less knowledgeable than you
- Do things that give you a sense of meaning, purpose and joy in life.

1. Focusing on purpose and meaning in life

As we discussed earlier, although our drive system can be a wonderful source of energy, focus and achievement, if it is overly directed by self-interest, competition or the avoidance of unpleasant feelings (e.g. shame, inferiority), this can be a source of distress and suffering. However, if we can guide the drive system by the motives of compassion, and balance it with the grounding experience of the soothing system, we might be able to benefit from its energy, directedness and vitality that come with it. There are two areas that we will focus on here: imagining a 'future' self, and clarifying what would be important in our lives.

Exercise 1: Imaging Our Future 'Best Possible Self'

Spend a few moments grounding yourself in your breathing rhythm. Sit in an upright, confident posture, allowing your facial muscles to relax. When you feel ready, spend five minutes imagining a future in which you are your *best possible self*. This is a future where things have worked out as well as they could for you, where you have worked hard, and experience a sense of purpose and meaning in life. Try to stay away from unrealistic or impossible goals or accomplishments, but focus instead on things that are realistic, positive and achievable. Imagine how you would feel, how you would think about yourself, if this future were possible. It might be helpful to focus on the following aspects of your life:

Relationships: Think about how you would like your relationships to be – with friends, family, and romantic partners. Spend some time imagining what your goals will be in these areas, and how you would like your social and family life to be.

Professional life: Think about how you would like your professional life to be – what sort of work you might be doing, the pleasure you would take from this, the goals you would have accomplished.

Personal: Think about how you would be, and the qualities and attributes you would have. How would you bring these into the world and to other people around you?

Really try to imagine these different aspects in detail – how you would be, how you would feel, and how you would talk, and interact with people. Now see if you can take a moment and describe in writing, and in as much detail as possible, your ideal future. You can use the categories above as a guide. Try to spend at least ten minutes on this (use a blank sheet of paper if you need more space). If you find this difficult, take a look at the 'hints and tips' section below.

Self-reflection: My ideal future

_____

_____

_____

_____

**Box 11.3: Some tips to help with becoming aware of competitive,
or threat-based drive goals, values and motives**

Tips – becoming aware of competitive or threat-based drive goals, values and motives

As you engage in the practices in this chapter, it's important to be aware of the motives, values or goals that sit underneath your drive system. As we explored above, although competition and the desire to 'win' are natural motives, it is important to become aware if and when these motives come with a sense of fear, conditionality, or a need to avoid pain (e.g. unless I achieve, I'm no good, others won't like me, etc.). This would indicate that our threat system is activated, rather than us engaging in things because we personally find them enjoyable and interesting (what is commonly often referred to as 'intrinsic motivation'). In fact, being overly competitive, relentlessly striving, and generally driven in a way that is guided by fear or anger can often lead to anxiety, distress, exhaustion and burnout. Some examples of this type of striving are:

- A drive to acquire money, objects (e.g. clothes, cars) to highlight our status or attractiveness

- A desire to be better than, or beat others

- A desire to exploit or take advantage of those less successful

- A desire to succeed, to avoid something unpleasant – for example, rejection, feeling like a failure or inferior

This is not to suggest that the above examples are bad or wrong, but may help you consider what is guiding your drive system. To minimise threat-system activation we will approach the following exercises by first helping you to ground yourself in the soothing system before connecting with your drive system (see Box 11.2, page 151, for hints and tips).

Valued directions – doing things that matter to you

Another way of orientating our minds towards our drive system is through clarifying our values. When we talk about values here, we are referring to things in our lives that matter to us, and bring meaning and a sense of purpose. Values are sometimes mixed with goals. Goals are things we can achieve and 'strike off', such as getting a new job, or running a half-marathon. Values, on the other hand, are more of a direction we continue to travel in (like north on the compass). Whilst they also involve action and sometimes a sense of achievement, they are centred more on the intention and direction of travel, rather than just the outcome (e.g. getting there / achieving it). In other words, the 'journey' or behaviours that take us toward something we value are rewarding in themselves rather than the end result on its own.

Whilst goals are important, we see values as useful in shaping and sustaining our drive system in a healthy way. We will therefore focus on how values, particularly those related to compassion, and qualities of empathy, sensitivity, motivation for wellbeing, and so forth, can inform, guide and support our drive system (have a look back at Chapter 5, pages 69–88, if you want a reminder of the qualities of compassion).

A benefit of being clear in our values is that we can identify and engage in the behaviours that are congruent with them, even if our threat system is activated. In a sense we can consider how we could lead a meaningful life, even if we feel distressed, low in mood or anxious. Let's take a look at a few examples:

Example1: Elijah had been feeling depressed for three months. He described feeling demotivated and struggling to enjoy things he would usually do, and for the past few weeks had stopped socialising and going to the cinema. However, although worried about how he was feeling, he continued to volunteer at the local homeless charity shop, as supporting people who were less fortunate than himself had always been important to him.

Example 2: Anne and her husband Harold wanted to start taking care of their physical wellbeing. Both were overweight and Harold had recently been diagnosed with diabetes. They were informed that the diabetes could be controlled by changing his diet and leading a healthier lifestyle. Both had tried dieting and exercise before, but always struggled as they enjoyed eating and drinking wine so much. However, they knew that their behaviour needed to become consistent with what they valued (each other and their physical wellbeing). They were also able to focus on their desire for fun, play and great holidays into their old age, and to spend time with their new granddaughter, Clara. They decided to embark on an active journey of self-care involving healthy eating and exercise.

Example 3: Karen experienced a lot of shame about her body. When she was fifteen she had emergency surgery, which left her with noticeable scars on her legs. Throughout her adult years she always covered her legs by wearing trousers, or long skirts. Although she dreaded it, more recently she was able to wear a swimming costume (thus showing her legs) and go to the beach to celebrate her niece's birthday, a child who loved building sandcastles. Karen's care and commitment towards her niece, and her valuing of spending time with her, enabled her to face what was otherwise a difficult task.

With these examples in mind, we would like you to think about your own valued direction in life. What things in life bring you a sense of inner pleasure and reward? Consider things that you would be willing to do, even in the face of low mood, shame or anxiety, because they hold an intrinsic importance to you, they matter to you and bring meaning and purpose to your life, rather than things that just 'feel nice' when they happen. To help you think about this, we developed Worksheet 11.1 overleaf, which you can complete. Think about what qualities you most value in your relationships, and the kind of person you want to become. You will see that there are separate sections for different areas of your life, such as home, family, work, social life, personal development and health.

Worksheet 11.1: Clarifying my values

Clarifying my values			
	What is my intention in this area? What do I value in this area?	On a scale of 0–10 rate how important this is in your life.	What would help me move towards my valued aims in the long and short term?
Working life			
Family life			
Friends and social life			
Personal development (e.g. education, skills, learning)			
Self-care, health and fitness			

Self-reflection: What was it like to spend time reflecting on your values? What did you learn about yourself?

_____

_____

_____

Given your developing skills in mindfulness and the soothing-affiliative system, how could these guide your values in a helpful way?

_____

_____

_____

Given what you've learned, consider what would bring you more in line with your values. What is your intention (what would you like to do) in the coming weeks with these in mind?

_____

_____

_____

Difficulties cultivating the drive system

As with many of the practices and reflection points in this book, it can sometimes be difficult to engage in behaviours, even though you recognise these would be in keeping with your values. If this is the case, have a read through Box 11.4 overleaf which outlines some of the most common challenges people commonly experience, and contains some hints and tips that might help.

Box 11.4: Common difficulties and helpful hints for cultivating the drive system

Common difficulties	Helpful hints
I've tried some of these things before, but they didn't make me feel any better.	This might be the most common experience that people tell us about – and a distressing one to have had. Try to hold a few things in mind if you can: It often takes practice to experience the benefit from new behaviours and activities. Remember what it is like when you first learn to drive, or learn a new language. It can take a while before you feel you're making progress. Imagine what you might say to a friend if he/she said this or felt discouraged; how you would try to validate their difficulty, but also support and encourage them to keep on trying to engage in behaviours and activities that are in line with their values.
I don't have any energy.	Not having much energy will understandably make doing some of these exercises more challenging. Try not be too hard on yourself with this, but instead see where you can start, and what small steps you might take. Try to focus your energy and commitment on what you feel you can do, rather than what you can't. It might also help to look at your expectations, and consider whether they are currently too high or unrealistic, given what else is happening in your life. If so, it might be worth considering altering your expectations, such that change can become more likely and achievable.

I'm already doing a lot of things, and I'm constantly trying to achieve things and push myself further. I can't see how doing more will help me.	This is another common experience for many people. Our research has found that some people engage in the drive system (e.g. by striving to achieve) in order to avoid feelings of inferiority and shame (linked to the threat system). Although understandable, this type of motivation is often associated with higher levels of stress, anxiety and depression symptoms. If this is the case for you, or if you feel that you are doing too much anyway, it might be more important to prioritise focusing on cultivating your soothing-affiliative system. This may give you a greater sense of groundedness and inner stability, and an overall balance. You might then want to revisit your activities and consider which are linked to fear, and which are intrinsically motivating for you.

2. Gratitude and appreciation

For many of us, it can often feel much easier to pay attention to the negatives and pains of life, rather than the things that we feel appreciative of or grateful for. As we've emphasised throughout this book, this is not our fault. Our brains are naturally set up in such a way that we will prioritise potential threats over everything else (remember the example of the shopper on page 25). However, although this is a natural way that our brain works, it is important to remember the phrase 'What we focus on expands' and also 'We become what we pay attention to'.

So many of the threats that occupy our minds are distant – they exist in the past, or some time in the future. All we know for sure is what we have this in very moment. Maybe this is why it's called 'the present'– because it can be a gift to us! As we found out in Chapter 8, developing our skills in mindfulness can be a powerful way to become aware of when and how our minds become overly connected with threat-based thoughts, feelings and memories (see pages 101–19). Recently, researchers and clinicians have found that *gratitude*, and deliberately focusing on and paying attention to *positive experiences* may lead to a variety of benefits. Research also suggests that writing about things that we feel grateful for can lead to an increase in joy and happiness, and a greater optimism for the future. Over time, this can also lead to improved physical health and lower levels of depression.

Being aware of the things we appreciate in this way does not mean that we ignore all the pain in our lives; rather, this noticing can bring a bit more perspective and balance in how we feel. Of course, being appreciative involves more than the drive system; it can be a process whereby we connect with our humanity and life in an open-hearted way, thereby activating our soothing-affiliative system. The key here, as we explored at the beginning of this chapter, is to allow ourselves time and space to 'let in' the positive.

Exercise 2: Three Good Things

Take a few moments to connect with your soothing breathing (see pages 126–31). When you feel ready, see if you can look back over your day, and write down three 'good things' that happened. This could be a wide variety of things, such as having enjoyed a nice meal with a friend, being treated kindly by a shop assistant, having had a good night's sleep or even receiving a compliment from someone. It does not matter how big or small these things are, as long as they give you a sense of happiness, joy or excitement.

- _____

- _____

- _____

As the American neuroscientist Rick Hanson comments, our brains are like Teflon for positives, and Velcro for negatives. It is therefore important that we really invest time focusing on positive experiences, so that they have an opportunity to take root in our brains. To do this, we are going to spend some time exploring each of the positive experiences you identified above, one at a time.

Good Event 1: _____

What led to this good event happening?

_____

_____

How did this event leave you feeling? (Spend some time bringing the situation/event back to mind, in as much detail as you can.)

_____

_____

What could you do so that more of these events happen in the future?

_____

_____

Plan: Repeat this step for each of the three good events you noted down earlier for the day. Remember, the key is to try and give this exercise enough time and space so that it can embed itself in your mind. To help with this, it is important to repeat the 'good things' exercise over a period of a week, each day focusing the spotlight of your mind on three positive experiences. As with everything else, the more you practise this way of focusing, the more likely the positives are likely to 'stick' in the brain!

Chapter summary

In this chapter we took a closer look at our drive system and explored some ways of stimulating it in a way that can be helpful.

What we have learnt together	My personal reflections on the chapter
1. The drive-excitement system is an important source of pleasure and achievement. 2. There are different ways of stimulating our drive system, and different motives (e.g. fear avoidance, competition, connection and affiliation) can guide the activation of this system. 3. It can be helpful to be mindful of overly competitive or threat-based drives that may underpin the drive system, and try to connect with motives linked to compassion.	

DEVELOPING OUR COMPASSIONATE MIND

In the previous sections of this book we've been building an understanding of our minds, along with skills that to help us to manage some of the difficulties we commonly face in life. In previous chapters we particularly focused on how developing skills in mindfulness – and ways to bridge from threat into soothing and drive systems – may help us to better manage our threat systems. We've learned how we can become more aware of our minds, and rather than getting trapped in threat systems, we may be able to shift to a different pattern. These are the first steps towards laying the foundations for developing compassion. There are a variety of ways that we can help to develop a 'compassionate mind', and here we will start by using memory, imagination and acting techniques.

Before we move into this, it can be useful to clarify our motivation for why it is important to focus on this. As you might have recognised from what we've covered so far, motivation sits at the heart of compassion. Compassion is a motive that helps to organise the other faculties of our minds, such as our attention, thinking, behaviour and so forth, enabling us to engage with and alleviate difficulties in life. It is therefore important to clarify what your compassionate motivation is – what you are going to focus your compassionate mind on in the coming chapters. Let's explore this together.

Exercise 1: Compassion-based Motivation – Why Do I Want Things to be Different?

Sit in an upright and comfortable position, and take a moment to find your soothing rhythm breathing. When you feel ready, see if you can connect to what you really want for yourself, and your motivation and intention to grow your compassionate mind. From this perspective, take some time to reflect and make some notes on the following questions:

Self-reflection: Why is it important for you to become a compassionate person?

_____

_____

_____

What would you like your compassionate mind to help you change in your life?

_____

_____

_____

How would you like things to be for you in the future? How would you handle the things that cause you distress if you were guided by your compassionate mind?

_____

_____

_____

What might challenge you in developing your skills in compassion?

_____

_____

_____

How will you manage these challenges?

_____

_____

_____

How would you treat yourself differently if you had a more compassionate mind?

_____

_____

_____

How would you relate to other people if you were more compassionate? What qualities of compassion would you have as a compassionate version of yourself?

_____

_____

_____

Compassionate motivation: The 'Two Wolves' story

Sometimes art, music and literature can play a powerful role in stimulating our motivation. One short story in particular that gets to the heart of compassionate motivation is that of the 'two wolves', which is attributed to Native American folklore. The story goes like this:

One evening a grandfather was teaching his young grandson about the internal battle that each person faces. 'There are two wolves struggling inside each of us,' the old man said. 'One wolf is vengeful, angry, resentful, self-pitying and scared ... The other wolf is compassionate, faithful, hopeful, and caring ...'

The grandson sat thinking, then asked: 'Which wolf wins, Grandfather?'

His grandfather replied, 'The one you feed.'

Self-reflection: Take a moment to reflect on this story; consider how it relates to you, and to your compassionate motivation for things to be different in your life. Think about how you can feed your compassionate wolf – your compassionate self.

_____

_____

_____

Try to hold these reflections in mind as you read through the coming chapters. Key is focusing on your motivation, with an understanding that, just like developing any skills in life, this may take practice, patience and persistence.

12 Developing our compassionate self

'Yesterday I was clever so I wanted to change the world. Today I am wise, so I am changing myself.'

– Rumi

In this chapter we are going to start the process of developing your 'compassionate self'. A useful way of understanding this is to recognise that rather than being made up of 'one' uniform and static self, we are made up of 'multiple selves'. Another way of saying this is that we have many parts of us, and these parts may operate in quite different ways from each other. For example, if you are shouted at by your boss in a meeting with colleagues, there may be an angry part of you that would like to shout back, telling them what you think of them and their (lack of) leadership skills. But in this situation there may also be an anxious part of you, which wants to disappear, run away and not attend any meetings again. There could even be a sad part of you that feels very distressed and tearful about the criticism, which wants to curl up and cry. If we are lucky enough, these parts are well integrated and we can experience all of them in a healthy, balanced way. We may even be able to connect with a part of us that is strong and grounded enough to tolerate our boss's criticism, wise enough to understand why he or she is reacting like this (e.g. that they are having a difficult time in life following the recent death of their mum), and committed to both finding a helpful way of sticking up for ourselves (e.g. speaking to our boss after the meeting, and sharing our feelings in an assertive but helpful manner about how their criticism was unhelpful in the way it was given in the meeting). From a Compassionate Mind Training (CMT) perspective, we would describe this part as our 'compassionate self', and in this chapter we are going to spend time together learning more about the qualities this part has, and crucially, how we can go about developing it.

Compassion as a self-identity

One way we can understand the concept of developing our compassionate self is to think about this as an *identity*. We can have multiple identities (for example, our gender, faith, job, nationality) or aspects of our personality (such as having a sense that we are an outgoing/ shy/funny person). Just as these identities influence how we think, feel and act in the world, when we develop a compassionate identity this also shapes aspects of our mind. Why is this important? Well, there is now a growing research literature suggesting that developing a compassionate identity and intention – and thinking, behaving and relating to people from this identity – can bring about significant changes in your life. These include engaging in compassionate behaviours towards others, feeling close to and supported by others, and experiencing lower levels of self-criticism, low mood and stress. We will explore specific ways of developing your compassionate self below.

Cultivating the compassionate self

Holding on to the idea of compassion as an identity, we're going to practise a number of exercises that help to cultivate this. In many ways, working on these involves developing a 'mind within a mind' – a part or version of us that thinks, behaves, pays attention to, and is motivated by a compassionate intention. A part of us that is sensitive to our own and others' suffering, and has a desire to do something about it, to reduce distress and prevent it returning. Even if you don't feel that you have a compassionate part in you, that's OK. These exercises are designed to help you develop this.

Developing your compassionate self – Acting techniques

It might seem a little strange, but one of the ways that we can help you to develop your compassionate self is through using techniques that actors are taught, and trained in. So this next part of the book is going to give you a chance to tap into your inner Robert De Niro or Scarlett Johansson!

So what can we learn from actors' training? Actors have to find ways to develop certain ways of being (thinking, feeling, behaving, moving, interacting, etc.) that best represent the character they are portraying in a way that is felt to be real and believable. And whilst the actor may have some lived experience or similarities to the particular character he or she is playing, quite often they don't. In these instances it is through the use of a variety of skills – including those involving memory, empathy, imagination, observation and embodiment – that they are able to 'step into' the state of mind of the person or situation they are playing. Often they closely study not only the history of the characters they are playing, but also their physical characteristics, such as body posture, facial expressions, tone of voice and behaviour. They also consider what it would feel like to be this character, and how they might see the world, other people and themselves through his or her eyes.

The crucial point here is the importance of creating space to practise *being the person you want to be* – to develop a compassionate identity, a 'compassionate mind' within your mind. There are a number of ways that we can do this, and will explore these together throughout the remainder of the chapter.

Using memory

A good way to start developing your compassionate self is to connect with the memory of what it was like when you were in this mind state in the past. In the scientific literature there have been thousands of studies investigating how memories are made, how they are recalled, and the impact they have on our feelings when we bring them back into our awareness. What is clear is that when we spend time focusing on a memory, and in particular, an emotional memory, we are often left with the same feelings that we had at the time the memories were formed. So, for example, if we chose to focus our attention on a time in the past when we felt rather anxious (for example, before a job interview) or a time when we felt really sad (maybe the death of a loved one, or the end of a relationship), we would experience glimmers of the same feelings in the present. Similarly, if we brought to mind memories that are linked to positive emotions and feelings (for example, of a time when we felt really happy or excited) we would begin to feel those emotions now. And of course if we remembered a time when we felt compassionate towards someone (or something) we would begin to experience feelings, such as care, kindness, warmth, commitment and courage. Let's try this using the exercise overleaf.

Exercise 1: Compassionate Memory

Sit in an upright, comfortable position. Engage in your soothing rhythm breathing (see pages 126–31). Allow your breathing to slow a little, and gently rest your attention in the flow of breathing in, and breathing out. Stay with this for sixty seconds, or so. Allow your face to relax, and gently bring a warm or friendly expression to it.

When you feel ready, bring to mind a memory of a time that you remember feeling compassion for another person or perhaps an animal. It might be a time when you offered help to someone struggling with a difficulty at work, or in their relationship. It could be a time that you helped someone to carry his or her heavy bags on to the train, or looked after your poorly pet. Try to pick a memory in which the other person or animal wasn't in too much distress.

Within this memory, try to remember what your intention was towards this other being – what did you want for them? Spend thirty seconds focusing on this, trying to hold that intention in mind.

Now see if you can remember what your body language or facial expression was like. Consider how the way you were standing, the way you held your body, or the expression on your face conveyed your compassion or kindness towards the other person. If you can, reconnect to an echo of that feeling now. Try to remember the words you said, the tone of your voice, or what you did to show your compassionate intention. Again, just hold in mind all these characteristics, and how they conveyed your compassionate desire for this other being. If you find it difficult to remember any of these things specifically, just imagine what your facial expression, voice tone or intention was like.

Spend a couple more minutes focusing on the memory. When you are ready just let the memory fade and make some notes or write your answers to the questions in the space below.

Self-reflection: How did you find this exercise? What was it like to recall being compassionate to someone else? Could you remember how you went about trying to do this (e.g. your facial expression, voice tone or posture; what you said or did to help)?

_____

_____

_____

_____

Box 12.1: Common difficulties and helpful hints with the compassionate memory exercise

Common difficulties	Helpful hints
I can't remember a time when I was compassionate to anyone.	It can be frustrating and disappointing when this happens. So, if you can, see if you can engage briefly with your soothing breathing and with a warm tone of voice, reminding yourself that this is not your fault and doesn't make you a 'bad' person.
	Sometimes it is helpful to reflect on what might seem like unimportant or insignificant experiences; for example, memories of holding a door open for someone, or wishing someone a nice day, or even taking time out to look after, stroke or feed a pet. The key thing is to give yourself the opportunity to connect with the experience of being kind, caring and helpful, regardless of how big or small the gesture was.
I could bring a memory to mind, but then I became emotional (sad, angry, anxious), as I focused on the difficulties the person was facing.	This is a common difficulty. While the memory might connect us to compassion, it can also re-engage us with the distress experienced at the time, which in turn can activate our threat system in a way that takes over the exercise. If this happens, two things can be helpful:
	1. See if you can return to your mindfulness and soothing breathing (see pages 101–19 and 126–31), and when you feel more able, slowly return to the memory again when ready
	2. Pick a memory in which you were being compassionate, but the situation was less distressing and therefore activating of your threat system.

Developing our compassionate self

We're now ready to work on developing our compassionate self in a more specific way. To do this, we can integrate what we've just learnt from the compassionate memory exercise, and also consider what sort of qualities we'd like to embody if we were able to cultivate a compassionate version of ourselves in the future. Take a moment to think about this for yourself. If you were able to develop a compassionate part of you – a version of you that, at some stage in the future, would embody compassion for others and to yourself – what qualities would you have? Make a few notes below:

_____

_____

_____

_____

Three core qualities of our compassionate self

Alongside the qualities you've named above, we're also going to focus on three specific qualities that we see as central to helping to develop the compassionate self. These are:

- Wisdom

- Caring-commitment

- Strength and courage.

We will explore each of these in more detail below.

Wisdom

Wisdom in compassion is essential. 'Foolish' compassion is not very helpful! The founder of Compassion Focused Therapy, Professor Paul Gilbert, gives a nice example of unwise compassion: imagine that you are walking along a river on a summer's day, and you suddenly see someone fall in and struggle to stay afloat. In your compassionate, caring state you run towards them and then dive into the river. However, mid-dive, you realise: 'Oh no, I can't swim!' The problem here of course is that whilst your intention is to be compassionate (i.e.

to try and save the person who is drowning), without wisdom and an awareness that you can't swim, your compassionate action may result in not one but two people needing to be rescued. On the other hand, if wisdom was to guide your compassion here, you might inhibit your immediate desire to dive into the water, and instead phone the emergency services, or try to find something (a rope, or a piece of wood) to throw to the person in the river to help them out.

Here's another example: if you've ever been on a plane, it's likely you'll remember that, should the cabin lose pressure, the flight attendants advise you to put oxygen masks on yourself before putting them on your child. This is wise, rather than selfish, as trying to help others before ensuring that we can breathe could put us in danger (i.e. we might pass out), which won't be very helpful to anyone! Instead, putting on our own mask first would free us to tend to others.

The American psychologist Abraham Maslow said 'If you only have a hammer, you tend to see every problem as a nail.' Wisdom in compassion helps us to step back and recognise when in life it is helpful (and wise) to use the hammer, and when it is not. Wisdom as a quality of compassion within a Compassionate Mind Training (CMT) perspective is also rooted in an understanding linked to the ideas we explored in Chapters 1–4. It gives rise to an appreciation that we all just find ourselves here with a tricky brain that we did not choose, but that can keep us stuck in loops. Wisdom in compassion includes an understanding that we are socially shaped – that we do not choose the environment we are born into, or many of the experiences we have in life, but that they play a major role in shaping us. Wisdom also allows us to appreciate that life is hard; that as part of being alive we will suffer, we will lose loved ones, experience rejection and setbacks, get ill and eventually die. This is the reality of life. A connection with this can help us recognise the pain and suffering that all of us will experience, and an understanding that this is so because we are a biological species and therefore by our nature, we age, decay and die.

Wisdom linked to the definition of compassion holds these realities in mind, but also helps us to learn how to take responsibility for doing what we can about them. This may involve learning to step back from blaming our own difficulties on other people. It may also involve trying to work out and understand what would be helpful responses to difficulties that arise. Wisdom can help us to consider other ways that we may approach or deal with the difficulties we face in order to alleviate, or reduce the nature of our distress in some way.

Self-reflection: Is there a person you know who you see as 'wise'? How have they displayed or embodied this wisdom?

_____

_____

Have you experienced times when you felt wise, or your wisdom influenced your behaviour in a caring and compassionate way? If so, how did your wisdom show itself?

_____

_____

What helped you, at the time, to bring wisdom to a situation?

_____

_____

Caring-Commitment

Whilst wisdom is an essential quality of compassion, we do not wish this to be applied in a cold or detached way, but instead with care, warmth and kindness. As Mark Twain, the great American author of the *Adventures of Huckleberry Finn*, is reputed to have said: 'Kindness is the language which the deaf can hear and the blind can see.' However, kindness may only be one aspect that sits behind compassion. In fact, sometimes acting kindly can be associated with the desire to be liked by someone or to avoid being rejected. As we discussed in Chapter 5, at the heart of compassion is the evolved motive to be *caring for*. So, to help cultivate and develop your compassionate mind, we want to build it around a motivated, caring-commitment to others and yourself. This is likely to involve various aspects linked to the intention and desire to be caring, supportive and helpful. Commitment here also involves recognising that while many of our struggles may not be our fault, rather than turning away, avoiding or ignoring these, we can learn to take responsibility.

Self-reflection: Spend a few minutes thinking about compassion and about caring-commitment. What are your thoughts about caring-commitment as a quality of compassion? Is this something that you've experienced from others, or demonstrated/expressed to others? Can you remember how you, or others, showed caring-commitment? How would you show this in your voice tone, facial expression, posture or actions? What would you feel if you were committed to caring in this way?

_____

_____

_____

_____

Strength and courage

If compassion involves the commitment to be caring and engage in that suffering, it's likely this will bring us into contact with distress. Whether this involves being with a loved one who is dying from terminal cancer, or making sense of and working through past traumatic experiences, the qualities of strength and courage are crucial. To engage in distress and not be overwhelmed by it, we need to have a sense of inner confidence, authority, strength and courage. If you consider international figures that are often labelled as compassionate, such as Martin Luther King Jr or Nelson Mandela, they are often described as 'strong' or 'courageous'. Courage and strength in compassion are like the roots of a tree; they allow us to remain grounded, and to tolerate and even approach pain and suffering without being overwhelmed.

Self-reflection: Think about strength and courage as qualities of compassion. What thoughts come to mind? Have you observed people being compassionate who also embody strength? Has your compassion ever involved being strong and courageous? How might you stand, sit or move if you had a strength, confidence or authority to your compassion?

_____

_____

_____

_____

Compassionate self – Practice

We've had a chance to explore some of the core qualities of your compassionate self. Now we're going to focus on how we can integrate these with what we learnt from the 'compassionate memory' exercise earlier in the chapter (see page 170). To do this, we are going to practise two related, but slightly different exercises.

Exercise 2: Compassionate Self I

Sit in an upright but comfortable position. Try to adopt a grounded, confident posture in your chair. Engage in your soothing rhythm breathing and friendly facial expression (see pages 122–28). Allow your breathing to slow a little, and gently rest your attention in the flow of breathing in and breathing out. Stay with this for sixty seconds or so.

Now, like an actor getting into a role, you are going to use your imagination to create an outline of what you would be like as a deeply compassionate person. So, for a moment, think about the qualities you would have if this were the case. If it helps, take a moment to think about someone you know who is very compassionate. What are the qualities that make them a compassionate person? Remember, it doesn't matter whether you feel you are actually a compassionate person. The most important thing is to imagine that you have the qualities of a deeply compassionate person – you are stepping into this character, this version of you – just as actors do when they take on a role. Let's spend sixty seconds imagining these qualities.

We are now going to focus on the three specific qualities of compassion that we discussed earlier in the chapter – wisdom, strength and caring – commitment. We will focus on each one of these in turn.

The first quality of your compassionate self is wisdom. There are many sources of wisdom: one comes from an understanding that we have tricky brains, which often get caught up in loops, or strong emotions and desires, that are difficult to manage. We didn't choose to have a mind that works like this. In fact, so much of who we are – our genes, our gender, our ethnicity or culture – we did not choose either, but this has had a significant impact on the person we are today. If we'd been raised by our next-door neighbours, rather than in our house by our caregivers, we would be a different person today. So your compassionate self has a deep wisdom about the nature of life itself, knows that so many of our problems are rooted in things that have been beyond our control – that much of what goes on in our minds is not our fault.

The wisdom of your compassionate self is also linked to learning how to take responsibility for doing something about your suffering. This involves stepping back from blame, shame and judgement and cultivating our minds in a way that might be helpful. Just as the grass, flowers and shrubs of a garden can grow in all sorts of ways, if we want it to look different we need to spend time cultivating it. Our compassionate wisdom unfolds to help us learn and develop skills that help us alleviate the distress and difficulties we meet in life. Spend sixty seconds or so focusing on what it would be like to be a wise person.

Now, bring to mind the quality of strength and authority. This strength emerges from both the wisdom of understanding the reality of distress and suffering in life but also the commitment to do what we can about this. It involves courage to face difficulties and tolerate the discomfort they bring, as well as our fears about change. Imagine that your compassionate self is strong and has an inner confidence; feel this connected to your upright body posture, feet grounded on the floor and breathing rhythm. Consider what tone of voice you would use, how you might stand and walk as a strong, confident person. Spend a short time bringing to mind what it would be like to be a strong, confident, compassionate authority.

Finally, let's focus on the quality of commitment. Your compassionate self has a deep caring-commitment – this is partly linked to an appreciation that life can be very hard, and that we may all struggle with many things. So given this, your compassionate self is motivated to be caring, and committed to alleviate your own, and other people's, suffering. It also has a desire to contribute to your own, and other peoples, wellbeing. It recognises that while many of our struggles are not our fault, we can take responsibility for acting in ways that are helpful and wise. Imagine how you would stand if you had a connection with this. Consider what your facial expression, or your voice tone, might be like if you were deeply caring and committed to alleviating suffering. Spend sixty seconds on this.

Often, people find that practising this exercise regularly over a number of weeks helps with feeling more connected to the idea of the compassionate self. Try to imagine these qualities – caring-commitment, wisdom, strength – coming together into a sense of your compassionate self. Take sixty seconds or so imagining your compassionate self with these qualities. How might you stand, how might you speak? How would you think and feel? How would you try to respond to people as your compassionate self? Focus on the desire to think, behave and feel compassionately. Don't worry if you don't feel that you have these qualities. Like an actor playing a character, just imagine what it would be like if you did.

Spend a couple more minutes allowing yourself to connect to your compassionate self. Take your time on the different qualities. When you feel ready, just let the image fade, and make some notes, or write your reflections to the questions below.

Self-reflection: What was that exercise like for you? Were you able to connect with certain parts of your compassionate self more than others? If so, which were easier/harder for you?

_____

_____

_____

_____

We're now going to explore a variation of the above exercise, using our imagination to help us 'step into' being our compassionate self.

Exercise 3: Developing Your Compassionate Self – II

Sit in an upright but comfortable position. Try to adopt a grounded, confident position in your chair. Engage in your soothing rhythm breathing and friendly facial expression (see pages 122–28). Allow your breathing to slow a little, and gently rest your attention in the flow of breathing in, and breathing out. Stay with this for sixty seconds or so.

In this exercise we are going to ask you to imagine that you can see your 'compassionate self' in front of you, embodying certain qualities. This could be you as you see yourself in the mirror, or a version of you (i.e. an image resembling you with a few small differences). However, you may imagine your compassionate self as someone quite different to you – someone you feel embodies compassion (for example, a colleague, friend or someone you've seen on TV). We'll first spend some time reminding you of the core qualities of compassion that we focused on before – wisdom, strength and caring-commitment. Here, we will go through them one at a time.

The first quality of your compassionate self is wisdom. There are many sources of wisdom. One comes from an understanding that we have tricky brains that often get caught up in loops, or strong emotions and desires, and are difficult to control. We didn't choose to have a mind that works like this. In fact so much of who we are – our genes, our gender, our ethnicity or culture – we did not choose either, but this has had a significant effect on the person we are today. If we'd been raised by our next-door neighbours rather than in our house by our caregivers, we would be a different person today. So your compassionate self has a deep wisdom about the nature of life itself and knows that so many of our problems are rooted in things that have been beyond our control – that much of what goes on in our minds is not our fault.

The wisdom of your compassionate self is also linked to learning how to take responsibility for trying to do something about all of this suffering. This involves stepping back from blame, shame and judgement, and cultivating our minds in a way that might be helpful. So just as the grass, flowers and shrubs of a garden can grow in all sorts of ways if left to themselves, the wisdom of your compassionate self can help you appreciate that if the version of you is not how you would like it to be – if it is contributing to your or others' distress – that you can do something to change things.

Now, bring to mind the quality of strength and authority. This strength emerges from both the wisdom of understanding the reality of distress and suffering in life, but also the commitment we have to do what we can about this. It involves the courage to face difficulties and tolerate the discomfort they bring, as well as our fears about change. Imagine that your compassionate self is strong and has an inner confidence to it. Consider what tone of voice you would use, how you might stand and walk. Finally, let's focus on the quality of commitment. Your compassionate self has a deep caring-commitment. This is partly linked to an appreciation that life can be very hard. So given this, your compassionate self is motivated to be caring, and committed to alleviate your own, and other people's suffering. It also has a desire to contribute to your own, and other people's, wellbeing. Spend sixty seconds reflecting on this.

Take a moment now to imagine what your compassionate self (this committed, wise and strong character) would look like if you could see it in front of you – its height, appearance, maybe even the clothes it would wear. Spend thirty to sixty seconds doing this. This version of you might look quite similar to you, but it might be a little different (e.g. slightly taller or shorter, older or younger) or very different (e.g. a different person or gender).

Now take a few moments to consider aspects of its appearance and nature. Take thirty seconds on each:

- Imagine how your compassionate self might stand, given their commitment and strength

- Imagine what their facial expression would be, and how this would convey their wise, compassionate nature

- Imagine what their voice tone would sound like, and how this would convey their caring nature and strength.

When you have an outline of this image, and you can get a sense of this standing in front of you, imagine slowly moving towards it. Pay attention to its posture, facial expression and compassionate qualities. As you get closer to it, imagine now merging with it. Imagine stepping into the shoes of this image – your ideal compassionate self. You're now standing in the shoes of this compassionate version of you, in its body and posture, looking out of its eyes with motivation to be kind, caring and compassionate in the world. Notice how it feels to be embodying your ideal compassionate self, with their wisdom, caring-commitment and strength. If it helps, imagine walking in the body of your ideal compassionate self. Notice how you would hold your body, how you would move, your facial expression and posture as you move around as your compassionate self.

Spend some time trying your best to embody and connect with your ideal compassionate self. When you feel ready, slowly allow this image to fade away, and spend a moment tuning into your soothing breathing.

Self-reflection: How did you find this exercise? Was it similar or different to the previous one? How did stepping into the shoes of your compassionate self feel? What did your compassionate self look like? (For example, if it looked different to you, try and describe it here.)

_____

_____

_____

_____

As you develop and practise these exercises and become more confident in connecting with your compassionate self, you can start using this part of you to engage with various aspects of your life. We will return to this in the remaining chapters of this book, but for the time being, like any skill, it might be helpful to set your intention to practising these exercises as often as you can.

Box 12.1: Common Difficulties and Helpful Hints for Trying to Develop a 'Compassionate Self'

Common difficulties	Helpful hints
It's too hard to focus on all the different qualities – caring-commitment, wisdom and strength.	If you feel overwhelmed, take it in smaller chunks. Maybe you can start with one of the qualities first and then move on from there.
I can't imagine having these qualities – I couldn't even imagine my facial expression or body posture.	Again, try not to be too hard on yourself for this, or to feel too dispirited – it can be difficult learning new skills, and other people also struggle with this exercise too. However, keep on going if you can. If it helps, break down the qualities into smaller steps, and spend some time thinking about each one separately before moving on. Remember, like an actor taking on a role, it doesn't matter whether you feel you are a compassionate person, or have any of the qualities we've been discussing. It can be helpful to just consider what it would be like if you did have some of them.
What's the point? It's not real.	Whilst this exercise is using imagination, researchers have found that by practising imagining this version of you, it may actually change the way you think, feel and behave in life. It might be helpful to look back to Chapter 10 where we explored some of the concerns about imagery and why this can be a powerful way of impacting on your mind and body.
I can't do this at all – there must be something wrong with me.	Try to remember it's not your fault if you find this difficult. Often there are good reasons for why we struggle to practise these types of exercises, and it can be particularly difficult to practise developing your compassionate self if

you have a lot of distress in your life, or if you have had very little experience of compassion.

It can be helpful to look over the fears of compassion chapter (Chapter 25, pages 342–9) to see if you can understand your struggles.

Keep on trying. Although it's hard at the moment, it's likely that further practice will make things a little easier.

Box 12.2: Tips for the Practice of the Compassionate Self

Tips – practice of the compassionate self

- For many people, using imagery to develop their compassionate self is very powerful. Often, however, people find it helpful to bring their imagery into real life in whatever way they can. One way of doing this is to try to 'be' aspects of your imagery in real life. So, for example, rather than just imagining your posture, voice tone or the facial expression of your compassionate self, like an actor you could practise this for 'real'.

- It does not matter if you think that you do not actually possess these qualities, just focus on imagining what it would be like if you did have them.

- Every day imagine being this compassionate person, practising voice tone, facial expression and compassionate body posture. If you feel that you do not have the time to practise the exercises then just remind yourself that little and often is OK. Just try and spend a few minutes focusing on your desire to be wise and compassionate, reminding yourself that you have the ability to be courageous and strong. You can practise as you brush your teeth, whilst lying in bed or in the bath, sitting in a waiting room or even on the way home from work. Remember, small changes can add up to make a big difference.

- It is sometimes helpful to find active ways of developing your compassionate self further. If this is the case, it may be helpful to move to Chapter 15 (pages 197–206), as this focuses on further developing your compassionate self by focusing it on other people.

Chapter summary

In this chapter we've focused on how we can develop our 'compassionate self' – a part of us that is wise, strong and committed.

What we have learnt together	My personal reflections on the chapter

1. Like other attributes and skills, we can spend time focusing on and practising to develop a compassionate part of us – our compassionate self.
 	
2. Our compassionate self may have many qualities. Three core qualities are:
 	
   • Commitment
 	
   • Wisdom
 	
   • Strength.
 	
3. Just as actors manage to step into the shoes of different personas, we can also develop the compassionate part of ourselves through the use of memory, imagination, and by focusing on our physicality (i.e. body posture, facial expression, voice tone, etc.).	

13 Developing our compassionate other

'From the very first hours of our lives right through to our last moments, kindness, gentleness, warmth and compassion are the things that can sustain us and help us bear the setbacks, tragedies and suffering that life will rain on us.'

– *Paul Gilbert, The Compassionate Mind*

In the previous chapter we explored how, by using memory, imagination and acting techniques, we could develop our compassionate self – a part or version of us that is wise, strong and committed. We discussed how we could see this practice as a way of developing a new type of 'mind within our mind'. In this chapter we're going to extend this work by developing an image of a compassionate 'other' – an image of another being that is committed to us and has compassionate qualities of wisdom, commitment and strength. If you remember from Chapter 10 when we developed an image of a safe place, we learnt that imagery can have a powerful effect in helping us to feel calm, safe and at ease (see pages 134–46). The same principle applies to creating an image of a compassionate other. Our brain and body can respond to the image of a warm, caring and compassionate being in similar ways to if a real person was treating us this way. This type of practice has been used over thousands of years in different religious and spiritual practices. Of course, you don't have to be religious or spiritual to benefit from it and we'll explore this together in the exercise below.

Creating an image of your ideal compassionate other

To start this process, it's useful to spend a moment thinking about what qualities of compassion you would like an ideal compassionate other to have. To do this, it could be helpful to spend a moment thinking about the following:

1. Bring to mind someone who has been compassionate towards you in the past. What qualities did they have? How did they convey their compassion to you? What personal characteristics or attributes did they have?

2. If you've seen someone show compassion to others, what qualities did they have? How did they show their compassion?

3. If you were having a tough time, what qualities would you find helpful in a person trying to support you?

Self-reflection: Spend some time noting down some of the qualities of compassion that the above scenarios brought to mind:

_____

_____

_____

_____

Just as we did in the last chapter when we focused on developing our compassionate self, here we want to build an image around three core qualities of compassion: wisdom, commitment and strength.

Wisdom – your ideal compassionate other is wise; they have a deep understanding about you, the difficulties you struggle with, and how you've tried to manage these. But they also have an understanding of the complexities of life and the suffering we can all face, that we all have tricky brains, that we have been shaped by evolution and/or social circumstances, and that much of this we didn't choose. The wisdom of your compassionate other also involves them having an understanding of what might help you to manage or cope with the difficulties you're facing.

Commitment – your ideal compassionate other is motivated to care for you – to help you deal with the difficulties you experience and to help you flourish and be happy in life. They are kind, understanding and supportive.

Strength – your ideal compassionate other has an inner strength and confidence; because they have an understanding of and commitment to you, they are able to be with and tolerate any distress you might have. Like an ancient tree with deep roots, they are stable, secure and grounded.

Sometimes people find it helpful to think about how they would like their image to be. To help with this, take a little time to reflect on the questions below.

Exercise 1: Thinking About Your Ideal Compassionate Other

What would you like your ideal caring, compassionate image/other to look like? Describe their physical appearance. Would you want your ideal compassionate other to be human or non-human, for example an animal, or a part of nature?

_____

_____

How would you like your ideal compassionate other to sound? What compassionate tone of voice would they have? Would it be soothing, calm, soft or strong?

_____

_____

How would you like your ideal compassionate other to relate to you? Would anything help you to sense their commitment and kindness to you?

_____

_____

Imagine their facial expressions. Are they smiling? How are they showing concern for you?

_____

_____

How would you like to relate to your ideal compassionate other?

_____

_____

We're now going to spend some time using imagery to create an outline of your compassionate other. Try to remember that, just as with previous imagery exercises, images can often be fleeting and hazy, and rarely like a Polaroid picture. Try the exercise below, taking your time to develop and explore your ideal compassionate other.

Exercise 2: Creating Your Ideal Compassionate Other

Sit in an upright but comfortable position. Engage in your soothing rhythm breathing and friendly facial expression (see pages 122–28). Allow your breathing to slow a little, and gently rest your attention on the flow of breathing in, and breathing out. Stay with this for sixty seconds or so.

Take thirty seconds to bring to mind some of the qualities of compassion you would value in another. For the purposes of this exercise, we will guide your image around the following three qualities:

Your ideal compassionate other is *wise*: They have an understanding about the nature of suffering, that we have 'tricky brains', and recognise that much of what happens inside of us is 'not our fault'. They understand the difficulties we experience in life, and are able to offer helpful perspectives on this.

Your ideal compassionate other is *strong and courageous*. They have a sense of authority and quiet confidence to them, and are able to tolerate your distress and difficulties. No matter what, they will always be there for you, offering their support and strength.

Caring motivation: Your ideal compassionate other will have a deep caring-commitment to you. It is there to support and to help you. It does not criticise you but wants to help you to build compassion for yourself, and for other people. Whilst it understands that your struggles are not your fault, it wants to help you find ways of taking responsibility for your difficulties and find ways to act that are helpful and supportive.

With these qualities in mind – wisdom, strength and caring-commitment – what would your ideal compassionate other look like? Spend a few moments imagining this. Maybe you could consider whether they are old or young, male or female, short or tall. Perhaps your image isn't human – it could be an animal or part of nature – again, pay attention to what this image looks like. Spend a minute just allowing your mind to bring an image into focus.

How would you like your ideal compassionate other to sound? If they have a voice, what would their tone of voice be like? Spend a little time imagining this, and focusing on how the voice tone leaves you feeling.

If your image has a face, what's their facial expression like? How does their face express their compassionate nature?

How would you like your ideal compassionate other to relate to you? Would anything help you to sense their commitment and kindness to you?

It may be helpful to consider how your ideal compassionate other became compassionate – maybe they have experienced pain and suffering, but learnt how to dedicate themselves to the compassionate path. They understand the reality of pain and suffering that is part of life.

Your ideal compassionate other wants to be there just for you. They offer you their strength, wisdom, understanding and support. *What does it feel like, knowing that this ideal compassionate other is committed to supporting you?*

Spend a couple more minutes thinking about the image. When you are ready, just let the image fade and make some notes, or write down your reflections to the questions below.

Self-reflection: How did you find this exercise? How did if feel to create an image of a compassionate other? What was it like to receive its wisdom, strength and care?

_____

_____

_____

_____

What did your compassionate other look like? Try and describe its physical qualities – for example, age, gender, facial expression or voice tone.

_____

_____

_____

Difficulties imagining an ideal compassionate other

It's common for people to find aspects of this exercise a little tricky or anxiety provoking. Let's have a look at some potential obstacles, and some ideas as to what could support this process.

Box 13.1: Common difficulties and helpful hints for the 'ideal compassionate other' exercise

Common difficulties	Helpful hints
I couldn't get a clear image of anything.	Try not to worry too much if this is the case. It's quite common to find it difficult to get a clear image. The most important thing is to try and focus on the compassionate intention that your ideal compassionate other has for you, and to practise being open to receiving this.
I created an image, but it felt uncomfortable to think about it having compassion for me.	There can be many reasons why people find receiving compassion difficult – it might be helpful to look through Chapter 7 again on the fears of compassion from others (see pages 94–98). You may also find it helpful to read Chapter 25 (pages 342–49), which explores how we can manage common difficulties and blocks to compassion.
I want somebody that is real to care for me, not an imaginary person.	This is a very understandable feeling, and we also want you to have real people in your life to care and support you. We are not suggesting that your compassionate other should replace real people. However, sometimes it is hard to experience kindness and compassion from people, or to know what this is like. Your ideal compassionate other can help you to begin to experience these qualities from another and use them to manage your distress. This can support you to gradually move towards 'real' people and develop the type of connections and relationships you would like. At this stage, what matters is experiencing the intention and the feeling of being cared for and supported, rather than whether this comes from a real person or not.

As with the exercises in the previous chapters, it's usually helpful to dedicate time to practising and developing the image of your compassionate other. It may help to set your intention for when you practise this exercise in the coming days and weeks.

Chapter summary

In this chapter we've continued to work on developing our compassionate minds, this time through developing an image of an ideal compassionate other. In the coming sections of the workbook we're going to look at how we can use and direct your compassionate mind to help you engage with difficulties in your life, and find ways to alleviate your distress.

What we have learnt together	My personal reflections on the chapter
1. We can use imagery to create an ideal compassionate other who has certain compassionate qualities – wisdom, strength and commitment to you. 2. The image can help you to experience compassion from 'another' being. 3. There can be certain common difficulties when starting to practise this exercise, which we can work on overcoming.	

14 Developing our compassionate team

'No one can whistle a symphony. It takes a whole orchestra to play it.'

– H. E. Lucock

In the previous two chapters we have been focusing on developing two core practices that form the foundations of our compassionate minds: our compassionate self, and our ideal compassionate other. In this chapter we are going to explore how it feels to bring these together in a way that might further give you a sense of strength, courage and support. There are parallels here to the scientific literature, where researchers have found that people tend to have lower levels of distress, fewer mental health problems and higher levels of wellbeing when they (1) feel that they can turn to other people for support, reassurance, care and encouragement, and (2) when they are not with other people can turn inwards and experience those same qualities internally – inner support, reassurance, care and encouragement for oneself.

In this next exercise we are going to imagine our compassionate self meeting our compassionate other, and working together to support you.

Exercise 1: Developing Your Compassionate Team

Sit in an upright position, and just allow your muscles to relax and your mouth to make a gentle smile. Engage in your soothing rhythm breathing and friendly facial expression (see pages 122–28). Allow your breathing to slow a little, and gently rest your attention in the flow of breathing in, and breathing out. Stay with this for sixty seconds or so and then bring to mind the qualities of your compassionate self – caring motivation, wisdom, and strength.

Imagine walking along a beautiful path, or maybe through your safe place, as your compassionate self. Notice your body posture, facial expression and voice tone. Imagine that in front of you, you can begin to see the image of your ideal compassionate other. You know that your ideal compassionate other has a deep caring-commitment towards you and your compassionate self. Try to hold in mind that your ideal compassionate other has a deep wisdom about the nature of life, but also of your compassionate self – it appreciates its motivation and intention to be supportive and compassionate to you, and to other people.

As your compassionate self, notice the features of your ideal compassionate other – its facial expression, body posture and voice tone. Notice its desire to want to support you, to lend its strength, wisdom and motivation to help you. Notice how this feels for your compassionate self – to know they are supported by someone, or something, else. Take a moment to take pleasure in how this feels for the compassionate self – to know that it has the support and caring-commitment of your ideal compassionate other.

Spend a moment to focus on how it feels to be part of a team – a team which has a deep motivation, strength and wisdom, and which is keen on helping you to cope with the difficulties you might face in life. As your compassionate self, imagine that your ideal compassionate other is now stood alongside you – that, shoulder to shoulder, you are joined, supporting each other and looking outwards to the world with caring-motivation, strength and wisdom.

Remember, you can return this exercise at any time you wish. Spend a couple more minutes thinking about the exercise, making your facial expressions as compassionate as you can. When you are ready, just let the memory fade and make some notes or write your answers to the questions in the spaces below.

Self-reflection: How did that exercise feel for you? What was it like to imagine your compassionate self, and ideal compassionate other, meeting and supporting each other?

_____

_____

_____

_____

_____

How does it feel to know that your compassionate self and compassionate other can work together to support each other and you?

_____

_____

_____

_____

How might you use this imagery exercise to help develop a sense of a secure base – a sense of groundedness, support and strength? Can you use this exercise to help you engage with important things in your life?

_____

_____

_____

_____

Chapter summary

In this chapter, we've brought together what we practised in the previous two chapters.

What we have learnt together	My personal reflections on the chapter
1. That we can imagine our compassionate self meeting our compassionate other, and that they can work together to support you. 2. That we can use the idea of a 'compassionate team' to help support ourselves with the difficulties we face in life.	

Section V

DIRECTING OUR COMPASSIONATE MIND:
Compassion as Flow

In the previous chapters we explored ways of cultivating our compassionate mind by developing our compassionate self and compassionate other. Practising these exercises over time helps to build our capacity for compassion, which in turn can be helped by learning how we can direct these skills in particular ways. You may recall that earlier in the book we introduced the idea of compassion as a flow (Chapter 6, pages 89–93). Just to remind you again, these are:

1. *Compassion flowing out*: Paying attention to the needs and feelings of others, and directing our concern and desire to be helpful to others (compassion for others)

2. *Compassion flowing in*: The experience of paying attention to, and to receiving and accepting the compassion of others to us (compassion from others)

3. *Compassion to ourselves*: Paying attention to and engaging our own feelings and needs, in order to find ways to try and be self-supportive and alleviate our own difficulties (self-compassion).

If you're feeling unsure whether you'll be able to engage in each of these flows, try not to worry; these flows are built upon natural human motivations that at some stage you will have experienced or will have engaged in. Consider the first one, compassion for others. If you see an elderly person fall over and hurt themselves, what's the urge inside of you? Or if your friend or family member is upset or distressed after being treated unfairly by someone? That feeling of being moved by their distress and wanting to do something to help is an example of this first flow. And if you have children, this flow of care and compassion is likely to have emerged very quickly after the birth of your child.

What about the second flow? Being open to and receiving other people's compassion. Well, although you won't have remembered it, this would have been one of the first experiences you ever had – receiving compassion and care from your parents or caregivers. But take a moment to think about this flow later in life; maybe a time when you've been distressed and experiencing pain, and someone else has been there for you, supporting you and offering you help.

And finally, what about the third flow – self-compassion? Well, although we might not realise it at first, this is also something we naturally do, often without thinking. If you fall over and cut your arm on the floor, taking the time to clean the wound of dirt, and putting a plaster on it, is an act of self-compassion.

In the coming chapters we are going to explore exercises that help to strengthen your mind in each of these flows. Similarly to the exercises we've practised so far in the book, some of these may be easier than others, and you might find that one or two of the 'flows' are easier than others. That's absolutely normal; just take your time with these practices, remembering that you can use the mindfulness, breathing and imagery skills that you've developed in the earlier chapters to support yourself with this.

15 Compassion for others

'Be a rainbow in someone else's cloud.'

– Maya Angelou

As we discussed in Chapter 3 (see pages 32–4 and 40–4), our children – and those of most mammals – survive not by being strong, autonomous and independent, but rather, by being cared for: being fed, sheltered, protected and nurtured by others. Although we have innate motives to care for our young, we have evolved extended caring, in which we are able to form attachments to people across the lifespan, and care for people across age ranges. It turns out that fostering care-based feelings and intentions for other people (the desire for them to be happy, to be free of suffering and to flourish) isn't just good for them, it can also have a positive impact on us. Research is increasingly highlighting how being kind, compassionate and caring to other people can have significant positive effects upon our brains, bodies and wellbeing.

There are various exercises that can help to cultivate our compassionate minds towards other people. In this chapter we are going to practise three related but different exercises:

1. Recalling a memory of a time when you were compassionate to another person

2. Directing positive emotions – joy, warmth and kindness – to another person

3. Acts of kindness.

Take your time with each of these, creating space to practise them on various occasions in the coming days, weeks and months.

1. Compassionate memory

Memories can have a powerful influence on how we feel, and purposefully re-connecting with them can re-stimulate many of the same experiences that we had at the time the memory was formed. In Chapter 12 we recalled a memory of a time when you were compassionate to someone as a way to build your compassionate self. However, whilst that exercise was designed to help build towards your compassionate self, here we are going to use the following exercise to pay more attention to the flow of compassion from us to another person.

Exercise 1: Memory of Being Compassionate to Another

Sit in an upright and comfortable position. Engage in your soothing rhythm breathing and friendly facial expression (see pages 122–28). Allow your breathing to slow a little, and gently rest your attention in the flow of breathing in, and breathing out. Stay with this for sixty seconds or so.

Bring to mind a memory of a time when you were compassionate to someone. This could be someone you are close to, such as a friend or family member, but it might also be someone you don't know so well, or even a complete stranger. For this exercise, don't pick a time when the other person was experiencing too high a level of distress as this may overly stimulate your threat system, and block you from re-connecting to your experience of compassion.

Spend a few moments holding the memory in mind, trying to recall different details of it – where you were, what was happening, what you can see around you. Try to bring back to mind, or imagine, the motivation you had to be caring and compassionate to this other person. Now, try to recall how you showed your compassion to this person. How did you show it through your body posture, facial expression or voice tone? Spend a moment just holding in mind these physical qualities of your compassion.

Try to recall the words you said to the other person, and the intention you had for these to be reassuring, validating or helpful in some way.

How else did you show your care and concern? Maybe you did something to help the other person. Again, if you can, spend a minute or two holding in mind your desire to be helpful and kind – on the flow of compassion from you to the other person.

When you feel ready, allow this memory to fade from your mind, and spend a little while tuning in to your soothing rhythm breathing again. See if you can make a few notes in the space below.

Self-reflection: How was that exercise for you? How did if feel remembering being compassionate to someone else?

_____

_____

_____

What did you do? How did you act? What did you say to them? How were you showing your care and concern?

_____

_____

_____

_____

Box 15.1: Common Difficulties and Helpful Hints for Compassionate Memory

Common difficulties	Helpful hints
I couldn't think of a time that I was compassionate to someone.	This can be quite distressing if it happens, and can sometimes leave us feeling ashamed or critical of ourselves. If you can: • Try to validate your distress – it is understandable to feel disappointed when we struggle with an exercise • You're not the only person who struggles with this; others do as well • Allow yourself a little more time to think about the past. Maybe there was a time that you were compassionate to someone, but at the moment, because your threat system has been activated, it's hard to think of it.
I had a memory that seemed helpful to start, but then I began to feel anxious/sad/angry.	There can be a number of things that can lead to this. Sometimes if we pick a memory of someone that we have mixed feelings about (i.e. we care for them, but are also feeling quite angry with them at the moment as well), this can cause us

to feel angry during the practice itself. Other times, if the memory we have picked holds a lot of pain and distress (i.e. the other person's suffering was severe), although we may have had compassion at the time, we can quickly become threatened and overwhelmed by the distress and pain.

It might be helpful to focus this exercise on a different memory – or even a different person – one with a less threat-activating aspect.

2. Directing positive emotions and intent towards others

Another way of stimulating our compassionate minds for other people is by directing positive feelings and intentions towards them. These types of exercises are actually very old and have been practised as part of various religious and spiritual traditions for thousands of years. They are often referred to as 'loving-kindness' exercises, and are common in many types of Buddhist meditations. However, you don't have to be religious or to feel spiritual to benefit, as this is a general mind training exercise. Here, we are going to do a slightly adapted version of this exercise, helping you to get into your compassionate self first, and then engaging in the exercise from that part of you.

Exercise 2: Directing Your Compassionate Self to Others

Sit in an upright and comfortable position. Engage in your soothing rhythm breathing and friendly facial expression (see pages 122–28). Allow your breathing to slow a little, and gently rest your attention in the flow of breathing in, and breathing out. Stay with this for sixty seconds or so. We are going to bring to mind different qualities of compassion that we have discussed – caring-commitment, wisdom and strength. We will focus on each one of these in turn.

Focus on what it would be like to have a deep sense of caring-commitment – to be motivated to be caring, and committed to alleviate your own, and other people's suffering. Imagine how you would stand if you had a connection with this intention. Consider what your facial expression, or your voice tone, might be like if you were deeply caring and committed to alleviating suffering. Spend thirty to sixty seconds on this.

Next, let's focus on the quality of wisdom. Here, imagine that your compassionate self has a deep understanding about the nature of suffering, and knows that much of what happens inside of us is 'not our fault' – rather, it is the result of how evolution has created 'tricky brains' and how we've been shaped by life experiences which can lead us to think, feel and act in certain ways.

Finally, for now bring to mind the quality of strength and courage – that your compassionate self is strong and has an inner confidence and authority to it. Imagine what this would feel like – how you would stand, how you would speak, how you would feel a sense of roundedness and inner security.

Now try to imagine bringing these together – how you might stand, how you might speak, how you would think and feel, how you would try to respond to people – as your compassionate self. If it helps, take some time to read through the guidelines for this again in Chapter 12 (see page 167).

Now, as your compassionate self, bring to mind someone (or something) you care about - someone that you would like to be happy and content in life. This could be your partner, friend, parent or sibling; it could even be your pet. Really focus on this person – imagining what they look like, their facial expression. Focus on the feelings of care, kindness and compassion that you have for them. Hold this person, along with the positive feeling and intention you have about them, in mind for thirty seconds.

When you feel you have connected with your intent towards this person you care about, hold them in your mind's eye, as if you can see them in front of you. Then repeat the following statement with a warm, inner tone of voice, leaving a short pause between each phrase.

> May you be well (say their name)
> May you be happy (say their name)
> May you be content (say their name)
> May you tolerate the difficulties and distress you face in life (say their name)

Slowly repeat these phrases either out loud or silently to yourself. Really focus on your desire for this to be the case. Even if you don't feel it's possible for the other person to experience these things, this exercise is about the desire, the hope that it could be like this for the person you're thinking about. You can change the phrases or add to them if you want to, as long as they have a similar focus – directing positive feelings and intentions towards the other person.

Picture the other person smiling or acknowledging your good wishes. Just take your time and focus on your genuine desire to send the wishes to the other person.

When you have finished, spend a few moments grounding yourself back into your soothing rhythm breathing.

Self-reflection: What was that exercise like? How does it feel, having a genuine desire for another being to be happy, well, and flourishing?

_____

_____

_____

_____

Sometimes when we practise this exercise, we can feel a sense of warmth, joy or happiness at the thought that the person we care for may experience happiness. However, at times we may feel sad that they don't experience much happiness in life, or anxious that they might not in the future. Use your mindfulness skills to notice and tolerate these feelings as they emerge, knowing that they are understandable, given your care about that person (see pages 110–11). Continue to practise this exercise, using your compassionate self to guide and contain the process.

Happiness and compassion for others – developing your practice

When practising these types of exercises for others, we can direct these positive feelings and intentions towards different types of people. Often it's helpful, as we have done above, to start with someone that we have a deep, positive feeling for – someone who makes us smile. We may then want to move on to a friend or family member, before then moving on to a stranger. After this, we can turn up the difficulty settings. For example, we can try and direct loving kindness to multiple people, even entire groups of people. We may even try and practise loving kindness for someone we don't like! As you might imagine, each of these steps can take quite a lot of time, and can be quite difficult but over time, you might want to spend time practising this exercise, and observe how it leaves you feeling in relation to other people.

Common difficulties with directing compassion outwards

Although some people find directing compassion to others much easier than directing it to themselves, there are still a number of common difficulties that can emerge when trying to achieve this. If you found directing compassion outwards difficult, have a look at Box 15.2 below, which lists some of the common difficulties that people have described to us, along with some hints and tips that might help.

Box 15.2: Common difficulties and helpful hints with directing compassion outwards

Common difficulties	Helpful hints
I'm always compassionate to others, but no one seems to appreciate it or like me.	This is an important issue that has sometimes been referred to as 'submissive compassion' – that is, we attempt to be compassionate and caring to others, but we have an underlying motivation to be liked, wanted or not rejected. Try to remember that what we are practising here is very different. If you can, tune into your compassionate self and its intention of being compassionate to others.
If I'm compassionate to others then they'll just take advantage of me.	This is a common fear of compassion, and it might be helpful to re-read Chapter 7, which goes into this more. It may also be helpful to remember the key qualities of compassion that we are working on developing here. Whilst being kind and caring are important, remember too that strength and wisdom are also key, and that these two qualities are helpful in making sure that your compassion is not taken advantage of. You will have the strength not to allow this, but also the wisdom to know when your compassion is appropriate to someone else, and when it is being exploited.

3. Bringing compassion into reality – Acts of compassion, kindness and care

So far in this chapter we've practised directing the flow of compassion from ourselves to others by using our memory and imagination. However, we can also strengthen this flow by engaging in certain types of behaviours – those that are kind, caring and compassionate. Acts of kindness (bringing happiness to others) are not only good for other people but are good for us too. Research shows that helping other people can improve our mood, reduce stress and provide a sense of meaning.

Acts of kindness can be small gestures, such as smiling, saying hello to someone or they could be giving a thoughtful present or taking the time to write a 'thinking of you' card. The British clinical psychologist Paul Gilbert quite simply sums it up as 'If you spread sunshine to others, it can brighten you up too.' In the next exercise we will think about small ways of expressing your compassionate self in the world.

Exercise 3: Compassionate Actions

Think about the following question: How can I act in a kind and compassionate way to people today/ this week? Place a tick next to any activity that you would be able to do.

- Smile and say hello to somebody
- Ask somebody how they are
- Ask somebody how their day has been
- Offer to make someone a drink
- Invite someone around for tea
- Visit somebody
- Write a card or letter to somebody who is having a tough time
- Send a text message to somebody you haven't seen for a while
- Praise somebody
- Give somebody a compliment
- Hold a door open for someone

You may wish to write your answers to the questions in Worksheet 15.1 below. Sometimes if we have a plan of action in writing we are more likely to stick to the plan.

Worksheet 15.1: Compassionate actions

Questions to ask yourself	
How can I take more interest in people today?	
How can I be helpful today? What compassionate qualities would I need?	
What type of kind or compassionate acts do I intend to do today?	

Plan: If you can do, use your compassionate self to guide your acts of kindness. So spend a few moments connecting with your sense of caring-commitment, wisdom and strength, and then from that part of you, consider what types of acts of kindness you would like to engage with over the coming day / week. After you have completed the 'act', try to help this stick in your mind by replaying it in your mind, or making a note of it in your phone or diary.

Chapter summary

Practising how to direct compassion for other people has been found to have benefits both for the person we are being compassionate to, but also ourselves as the person giving compassion. We've explored this in multiple ways in this chapter.

What we have learnt together	My personal reflections on the chapter
1. That we can use our memory and imagery to direct compassion to other people. 2. That we can direct both positive feelings and intentions (e.g. for others to be happy) and compassion (that others may tolerate their suffering). 3. That we can plan to engage in a variety of compassionate ways – for example, through 'acts of kindness'.	

16 Experiencing compassion from others

'Minds are like parachutes – they only function when open.'

– *Sir James Dewar*

In the previous chapter we started to practise directing compassion towards other people. In this chapter we will help you to open up to receiving care and compassion *from* others. The exercises in this section aim to stimulate areas of our brain that are responsive to the care, kindness and compassion of others. Research has found that the experience of being and feeling cared for can have profound effects upon our nervous system, helping to regulate our distress and allowing us to tolerate difficulties in life, and engage and explore the world with confidence.

1. Experiencing compassion flowing towards you – using your ideal compassionate other

You will remember from Chapter 13 that we spent time developing an image of your ideal compassionate other. This was an image of a real or imagined person or being that embodied wisdom, care and strength. If it helps, take a quick look back to that chapter, and the notes that you wrote after doing the exercise, to remind yourself of the image you generated (see pages 184–88). In some ways just practising this was a way of experiencing compassion flowing from the outside towards you. Although the compassionate other was a creation of your own mind, rather than real, your brain is still likely to have responded to the image in a very similar way to the real thing. Here, we are going to use this image again, but this time focus more specifically on the aspects of receiving care and compassion from it.

Exercise 1 – Receiving Compassion From Your Ideal Compassionate Other

Sit in an upright and comfortable position. Engage in your soothing rhythm breathing and friendly facial expression (see pages 122–28). Allow your breathing to slow a little and gently rest your attention in the flow of breathing in, and breathing out. Stay with this for sixty seconds or so.

Bring to mind the image of your ideal compassion other – a caring, wise and strong other who has a deep intention to support you. Spend sixty seconds imagining what this looks like – its body posture, facial expression and voice tone. Hold in mind that your ideal compassionate other knows that we all just find ourselves here, with our tricky brains. They understand that our thoughts and feelings can run riot within us, and that this is not our fault.

Your ideal compassionate other is grounded and strong. It has confidence, so you know it can tolerate the difficulties and stress you experience in life. It has a deep desire to support you, to understand you. Your ideal compassionate other wants you to be happy and to flourish in life.

How does it feel, knowing that this ideal compassionate other is committed to supporting you? Spend sixty seconds or so remaining open to this flow of care and compassion from your image.

Focusing on the facial expression, voice tone and intention of this compassionate other, imagine them saying the following things to you:

> May you be well (your name)
>
> May you be happy (your name)
>
> May you find the strength and courage to tolerate your difficulties in life (your name)

Really imagine that your ideal compassionate other is looking at you with kindness, and is genuinely wishing you well. They feel connected to you and their wishes are heartfelt. Imagine hearing these heartfelt wishes in their warm, caring voice tone.

You may want to change the content of these wishes in a way that they are relevant and useful to you. Some examples are:

> I'm here to support you (your name)
>
> I'm here to help you tolerate your difficulties (your name)
>
> I'm here to help you reduce your distress (your name)

Play around with these phrases, finding the words and the tone of voice that you can connect with. Remember, try your best to remain open to the support and care of your compassionate other.

Self-reflection: How did it feel to receive compassion from your ideal compassionate other?

_____

_____

_____

_____

What was it like to know that your compassionate other was there for you, understanding you and genuinely wanting to support you?

_____

_____

_____

_____

2. Being open to the care, compassion and kindness of people in daily life

Life can be rather busy, and it can be all too easy to get caught up in daily stresses and strains. Whilst common, and very understandable, an unfortunate consequence of this is that we miss natural moments of genuine kindness, care and compassion from other people. Think about it for a moment. You have had a difficult day at work, juggling lots of projects and an unsympathetic boss. Or, you've been trying – and mostly failing – to keep your three young children occupied, fed and clean throughout the day. You pop to the local shop to get a few things for the evening meal, and as you go to pay, there's a really long queue that seems to take forever. The person at the till is very apologetic for the wait, and is very friendly towards you. They help you to pack your bags and wish you a nice evening. How likely are you to notice these gestures? Are you able to remain open to their warmth, kindness and help? Well, maybe sometimes, but often, in these situations, our threat systems are activated in a way that we don't spot signals of kindness and care coming our way, and we miss a real opportunity for connection and affiliation (i.e. soothing system activation).

What can we do about this? Well, to begin with, it can be useful just to know that this happens to all of us from time to time, and it is not our fault. Knowing this also provides us with an opportunity to 'look out' for, notice and savour this moment. Take a moment to think back over the last day or two. Were there any moments when someone treated you with warmth, kindness or care that you didn't think much of at the time? If so, take a few minutes to bring the situation back to mind. Replay the memory, focusing on the situation and what the other person did or said that conveyed their kindness to you. See if you can also bring to mind both their actions and words, and their facial expression and voice tone. Take your time, allowing yourself to be open up to this experience.

Self-reflection: What did it feel like to bring to mind a time of someone treating you kindly?

_____

_____

It can also be helpful here to consider your intention regarding this in the future. Take a few moments to consider what might help you to be more likely to notice, and be open to, the kindness and care of people. What would make it more likely this will happen? What might help you remember and hold on to your intention with this?

It might also be that there are certain people in your life who are naturally very kind and caring but with whom you find it difficult to be open to receiving this from them. If this is the case, it might be helpful to consider what your intention might be for the future with them. Could you set yourself to being open to receiving your friend's kindness and care? If you normally find it difficult to accept and be open to the care and compassion of others, what might help you to do this in the coming days or weeks? Which skills from this workbook could you use to help yourself with this?

Although this might not be easy at first, in our experience practising being open to the care, kindness and compassion of others can have a significant effect on our sense of connection and closeness to others, and our confidence in managing difficulties in life.

Chapter summary

We've continued to explore the flow of compassion in this chapter, with a particular focus on paying attention and being open to the care, compassion and kindness of others.

What we have learnt together	My personal reflections on this chapter
1. We can use memories and imagery to experience feelings of compassion coming from others towards us.	
2. We can create an ideal compassionate other to help us to develop a compassionate self.	
3. We can use our compassionate self to help us with our intention to be open to compassion and care from others in the future.	

17 Self-compassion

'If your compassion does not include yourself, it is incomplete.'

— Jack Kornfield

In the previous two chapters we started the process of helping you experience compassion in different flows, using a variety of exercises. In this chapter we are going to focus our efforts on directing compassion to ourselves. This is commonly known as *self-compassion*. Whilst many of us feel at ease being compassionate to others, and even receiving compassion from others, bringing compassion to ourselves can often be tricky. In fact, rather than being compassionate to ourselves, in times of difficulty we often treat ourselves in unkind ways. We can get caught up in invalidating our distress, fighting or trying to block it out – we can try and ignore it or push it out of our minds. Sometimes we can become very critical with ourselves for struggling as we do. In all of these, we tend to treat ourselves in a way that we would be unlikely to do if it was to someone else who was struggling in a similar way. So it turns out that being compassionate to ourselves is often quite a challenge, and that for many of us, it takes practice to learn how to become compassionate with ourselves. To do this, we will focus here on two specific exercises, but will return to expand on these practices later in the book (Sections VI and VII, see pages 219–349).

1. Directing compassion to yourself – imagery

Directing compassion towards yourself involves becoming more sensitive to your own distress and suffering, and finding ways to alleviate this in a helpful way. We will start to explore this with the following exercise.

Exercise 1: Focusing the Compassionate Self on Yourself

Sit in an upright and comfortable position. Engage in your soothing rhythm breathing and friendly facial expression (see pages 122–28). Allow your breathing to slow a little, and gently rest your attention in the flow of breathing in, and breathing out. Stay with this for sixty seconds, or so.

Bring to mind some of the qualities of your ideal compassionate self. Firstly, consider the quality of *wisdom*. You understand that we have 'tricky brains' that we did not choose for ourselves, but were created over millions of years of evolution. Again, imagine how it would feel like to look out through the eyes of your compassionate self with a deep understanding of how hard life can be, and knowing that all human beings face struggles throughout life. Secondly, consider the quality of *strength and courage*. Your compassionate self has an inner strength and confidence to it – it is grounded and can tolerate distress. Notice how being strong and courageous feels in your body. How would you hold your body? How would you stand with a sense of confidence and strength? Finally, consider the quality of *caring motivation*, a deep desire to be kind, caring and supportive in the world. Imagine having these qualities and how it would feel in your body to have the intention to be caring. Consider what your body posture would be like and what your facial expression would look like. What would your tone of voice sound like?

Now, holding onto your motivation to be caring, your sense of wisdom and strength, imagine walking down a street and looking through the eyes of your compassionate self. You have a deep intention to be sensitive to suffering, a desire to try to be supportive and to alleviate distress. Really notice how this feels inside. Imagine how you would walk, what your facial expression would be like, what your voice tone would sound like.

Next, imagine that you can see in front of you an image of your usual self, the version of you that is in the world at present, on a daily basis. As your compassionate self, look out to this version of you with deep kindness and with a caring motivation. You have a deep desire that this version of you finds comfort and happiness. Spend a few moments imagining this.

As your compassionate self, keep on looking at and connecting with the 'usual you' with your understanding of how life can be hard and stressful at times, and that this version of you is trying his or her best to manage with this. See if you can connect with your empathy for this version of you. Again, spend a few moments staying with this.

Given your caring intention and deep understanding of this version of you, consider what your compassionate self may want to say, or do. You may want to imagine saying the following phrases out loud, with a warm and kind voice tone, focusing upon the intention to be supportive:

> May you be well
>
> May you be happy
>
> May you find the strength and courage to tolerate your difficulties in life.
>
> If you prefer, you could use the word 'I'. For example, *may I be well, may I be happy.* Perhaps try both and see which one you connect with more. Spend a couple more minutes with this experience. When you are ready, just let the image fade, and make some notes or consider the questions below.

Self-reflection: How did you find that exercise? What was directing compassion towards you like?

_____

_____

_____

_____

_____

Sometimes it can be helpful to adapt the above exercise a little, imagining that your compassionate self is looking at a version of you that is in distress in some way. This could be stresses or strains you experience on the long commute to work, or the difficulties you're having in a relationship (for example, with your boss or partner). It might be the struggle you face managing a physical or mental health problem. The key thing is to engage in the version of 'you' that is distressed, whilst doing this from a part of you that is wise, strong and caring.

2. Compassion in the mirror

As the title of this exercise suggests, one way we can practise self-compassion is by practising this in front of a mirror. This practice is built upon the work of Dr Nicola Petrocchi and his collaborators, who carried out some interesting research on this. In this study, participants were split into three groups. In the first group, participants repeated out loud a set of four compassionate phrases. In the second group, people repeated the same compassionate phrases whilst looking at themselves in a mirror. In the third group, participants only looked at themselves in a mirror. The researchers found that participants who repeated the phrases *whilst* looking in the mirror had the highest levels of positive emotions, and significantly lower levels of self-criticism after doing the practice.

Given these findings, and our experience of how people have benefited from this in therapy, we will outline how to practise this for yourself. It is worth noting that if looking at yourself in the mirror feels overwhelming, you might want to look at a recent picture of yourself or alternatively, use your smartphone camera to see a reflection of yourself.

Exercise 2: Compassion in the Mirror

Sit in an upright and comfortable position. Engage in your soothing rhythm breathing and friendly facial expression (see also pages 122–28). Allow your breathing to slow a little, and gently rest your attention in the flow of breathing in, and breathing out. Stay with this for sixty seconds, or so. Bring the qualities of your compassionate self to mind, feeling your way into a sense of caring motivation, wisdom and strength.

When you feel ready, embodying your compassionate self, and connected to your soothing rhythm breathing and friendly facial expression, look at yourself in the mirror. Spend a moment just taking in the reflection of you. If you can, notice how it feels to bring a gentle smile or friendly expression to your face. As your compassionate self, see if you can direct feelings of care, warmth and kindness to your reflection in the mirror.

When you feel ready, repeat the following four statements out loud, or silently in your own mind, through a warm, caring voice tone:

> May you be well (your name)
> May you be happy (your name)
> May you be safe (your name)
> May you find the strength and courage to tolerate your difficulties in life (your name)

Notice how it feels to direct these intentions, hopes and feelings towards yourself. Continue to spend some time looking at your reflection, continuing to direct warmth, care and compassion to yourself. When you feel ready, repeat the same phrases to yourself again.

Self-reflection: How did you find this exercise? What was it like to use a mirror, or a reflection of yourself to direct compassion to yourself?

_____

_____

_____

Although this exercise can feel a little awkward at first, it tends to get less so with practice, and for some people it can be quite moving. It may also lead to you having the intention to pay a different type of attention to your reflection as you go about your day-to-day life; maybe taking short pauses when you see yourself in the mirror, gently directing care and compassion to this.

Looking forward

As with the exercises in the previous chapters, the key is to try and practise them as regularly as you can. If you're able to, it can be useful to try and practise one of these each day. As you can probably imagine, these types of self-compassion exercises can be challenging for various reasons. If this is the case, it can be helpful to have a look at Chapter 25, where we explore a number of the key struggles people have with being compassionate with themselves, along with some helpful tips about how we may manage these (see pages 342–49).

Chapter summary

In the final chapter of this section of the workbook we've explored a number of ways in which we can start to direct compassion towards ourselves.

What we have learnt together	My personal reflections on the chapter
1. Many people find it difficult to treat their own pain and distress in the same kind and supportive way they would someone else's pain and distress. 2. We can learn to direct kindness and compassion to ourselves. 3. By using our compassionate self, we can imagine giving compassion to ourselves, either through imagery, or by looking at ourselves in a mirror.	

SECTION VI

DEVELOPING THE SKILLS OF OUR COMPASSIONATE MIND

In Section V we explored how we could direct your compassionate mind in three different flows. In this next section of the workbook, we're going to explore how we can express, or direct, our compassionate minds in a variety of ways. Rather than being an emotion, compassion is linked to the motives of care-giving and care-receiving. Motives organise our minds in a particular way. So when we are in a competitive state of mind, our attention, thinking, feelings and behaviour (amongst other things) are directed and textured in particular ways. Take a moment to think about this yourself. Bring to mind a time when you've been in a competitive mindset – maybe going for an interview for a job you really wanted, competing in a game, or in a quiz. It's likely that this motivation affected:

- What you paid attention to (for example, focusing on who you were competing with or the task itself)

- Your thoughts (for example, thinking about what you should do or say to be successful)

- How you felt (for example, excitement, enthusiasm, or even tension)

- What you did / the type of action you took (for example, engaging in certain game strategies, planning your performance, etc.).

Equally, when we are in a compassionate state of mind, our attention, thinking, feelings and behaviour are also organised in particular ways. It may be helpful to look at the diagram below to consider how the compassion motive organises our mind.

A Compassionate Mindset

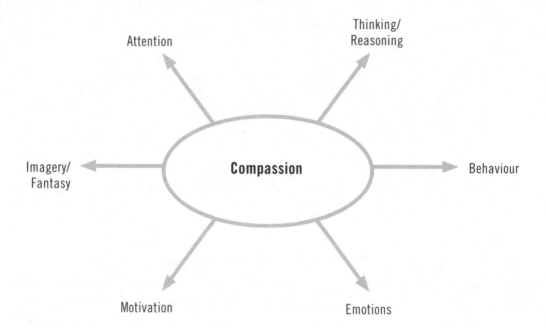

In the following chapters we will explore how we can further develop our compassionate minds through focusing more specifically on some of these areas. In particular, we will explore how to develop your skills in compassionate *attention, thinking, emotion* and *behaviour*.

18 Putting our compassionate mind to work – Compassionate attention

'The act of compassion starts with full attention.'

– Daniel Goleman

We have explored the nature of our attention at various stages of this book. We learnt that, like a spotlight, attention lights up what it 'shines' upon. We've also learnt that when the threat system is activated, this can capture or hijack attention so that we become overly focused on threats, difficulties and problems. While it is understandable why this happens as part of our evolved threat-protection system, it may not be compassionate to allow it free reign here. Consider the following example: you tell a joke at a party, and almost everyone laughs and seems to enjoy it. However, one person doesn't. After the party, your mind continues to focus on the facial expression of the person who didn't find your joke funny, and you begin to feel a lowering of your mood along with thoughts of 'I did something wrong. Why don't I ever learn just to keep a low profile?' So compassionate attention, as we will look at in more detail in this chapter, involves being aware of what our attention is focused on, and learning to be able to redirect it to something that might be helpful (for example, the faces of the people who did find the joke funny, or to other aspects of the party we enjoyed). We will explore this process in two key steps.

Step 1 – Paying attention to attention

A first step to developing skills in 'compassionate attention' is to understand what is happening with our attention in the present moment. To do this, it can be helpful to reflect on a few initial questions. For example, can I sustain my attention on the task that I'm engaged in? Does my attention tend to drift easily? If my attention does drift, what triggers this, and what does my attention go on to focus on?

To learn more about the nature of our attention, we can spend a few days monitoring it, making notes about what we tend to focus on, whether we become easily distracted, and what type of things tend to capture our attention.

Exercise 1: Attention Log

Monitoring attention can help deepen our understanding about its nature. It may be that some of us are very able to guide our attention in compassionate ways, but for others of us, it can be easy to become distracted (e.g. by mobile phones, email or noisy environments). Some of us might also find that our attention is captured by our threat system – for example, by something difficult that happened in the past, or by worries about things happening in the future. Worksheet 18.1 has been designed to help you monitor your attention and build your understanding. See if you can use this over the course of a day. Some people find it best to do this at the end of the day, looking back on various tasks they were engaged with over the day. Others find it difficult to recall this in detail at the end of the day, and prefer to complete it at more regular intervals during the day. The most important thing is to find a way to become more aware of what happens to your attention.

Worksheet 18.1: Attention Log

Time and date	What was I doing?	Where was my attention focused? Did anything (e.g. thoughts, worries, concerns) tend to hijack it?	How did what I was paying attention to influence my feelings?	If distracted, was it possible to redirect attention to focus on what I was initially doing?
Morning				
Afternoon				
Evening				
Night				

Self-reflection: Looking at your attention log, are you able to notice any patterns?

_____

_____

_____

Did you notice any common places your attention drifts to?

_____

_____

_____

How often did you find your attention was captured by (or was capturing) your threat system?

_____

_____

_____

As we learnt in Chapter 8, what we focus on (or pay attention to) plays our body. If our attention gets pulled into or captured by threat system-related content – for example, worries about the future, bad memories from the past, or negative thoughts about ourselves or others – we are likely to be left with a variety of unpleasant feelings (e.g. anxiety and anger). Remember, it is not our fault that our attention can get caught up in this way, this happens to everyone! This is part of the reality of having a 'tricky brain' that was designed for us, not by us. And if our attention frequently gets wrapped up in or captured by the threat system (whether the events we focus on are real or imagined), it is not surprising that we may begin to feel low in mood, anxious and unhappy in life. A challenge many of us face is *noticing* when this happens, as we are often unaware of when this has happened. Sometimes, when people complete this attention log, they find that attention gets hijacked by technology – for example, our mobile phones, social media and TV. When they look a little deeper at this, these types of distraction are sometimes used as a form of avoidance – to help us keep away from a threat system-related task (e.g. completing an essay or preparing for a difficult presentation or meeting).

So, what might help? Well, being aware that our minds can get caught by our threat systems could be a first positive step, and an example of the first psychology of compassion (i.e. being sensitive to, and engaging with our distress or suffering). This awareness can help give rise to the second psychology of compassion – taking helpful action to lessen our distress. We will explore this in more detail below.

Step 2 – Working with attention from your compassionate mind

So, how can we use our compassionate minds to guide our attention in a helpful way? Well, there are a number of things that might be useful here:

(i) *Mindfulness* – if you've spent time reading and practising the exercises in Chapter 8 (see pages 101–19), then you will have already started to work with your attention in a potentially helpful way. Remember, mindfulness involves paying attention in the present moment, without judgement. Learning to be mindful is learning how to bring our awareness to the here and now. But more broadly, mindfulness allows us to be more aware of what we're experiencing, while we're experiencing it – thus, mindfulness can help us notice when our minds (and in particular, our attention) is captured by the threat system, giving the potential for us to do something wise and helpful.

(ii) *Soothing rhythm breathing and safe place imagery* – using the body to calm the mind is a skill we've worked on throughout Chapters 9 and 10 of this book (see pages 120–48). Spending time practising your soothing breathing or safe place imagery may help to activate your soothing system. This is important because these exercises may help to engage our parasympathetic nervous system, which not only helps to contain the threat system but may also naturally stabilise our attention, making it less 'jumpy'. Let's have a look at an example.

Example: Edwin is getting ready to give a presentation to his colleagues later in the day. He has been looking forward to it because he will share some exciting findings from his research. However, prior to the presentation he begins to notice a little tension in his shoulders and stomach. This mindful awareness is followed by paying attention to his thoughts. Edwin notices thinking: 'What if my presentation goes horribly wrong? What if I blush in front of everyone, and make a fool of myself?' By paying attention to these inner experiences, Edwin recognises that his threat system is activated, and as a consequence he is left feeling anxious and wanting to avoid the presentation.

So, what helps Edwin here? Experienced at being mindful of his breath and body, thoughts and feelings, he uses this skill to notice the worry, anxiety and increased tension, and shallow breathing. He then re-directs his attention to his breathing and finds a soothing rhythm to help calm his body, and his mind. He also focuses his attention on what is around him – the feel of the ground under his feet, the breeze and sun on his skin – to help orientate himself to the here and now. Although worries about the presentation keep popping into his mind, Edwin continues noticing and directing his attention in the present, which eventually helps him to feel less anxious, and to concentrate on what he is going to do to get ready for the presentation.

(iii) *Learning what to pay attention to – directing attention in a compassionate and helpful way –* Whilst mindfulness helps to bring our attention to the here and now, it may also be useful to direct our attention in a compassionate way. This means focusing our attention on helpful alternatives, rather than leaving it at the mercy of our threat system. For example, if after giving a presentation our attention is grabbed by the threat system, replaying in our minds things that didn't go so well, we could use our attention to focus on things that are likely to calm and encourage us. Let's explore this using your own example:

Exercise: Consider a time recently when your attention was caught by your threat system. Maybe this was after a presentation, a meeting or a night out with a friend. Try to remember what your attention was getting caught up with, what you were focusing on, and what the threat thoughts or feelings were. Now, take a moment to sit in your upright, comfortable and confident posture. Engage in your soothing rhythm breathing (see pages 124–28) for thirty seconds or so, before spending some time connecting with the qualities of your compassionate mind. Through your compassionate mind, consider whether you can direct your attention to:

- An occasion during the event when things went well

- Moments in which you received positive feedback

- Previous occasions when you've managed these situations well

- Occasions in which others valued you, your work or company

- Memories of feeling appreciated and able.

With each of these, try to hold these moments in your attention in as much detail as you can. Rest your attention on each, focusing on the associated feelings these leave you with. This exercise isn't about trying to 'think positive', but rather an appreciation that the threat system narrows attention, making us focus on the negatives in a 'better safe than sorry' way. To counter this bias, we may need to purposefully focus on opening attention to create greater balance.

Self-reflection: What was this exercise like for you? What was it like to re-direct your attention in this way? How could you maintain this approach for the future?

_____

_____

_____

(iv) *Using our compassionate mind to see what is behind the focus of our threat attention* – as we discussed above, it can be helpful to become mindfully aware of what pulls our attention, use skills to notice this, and gently return our attention to refocus on what we are doing in the present. Whilst the above steps can be very helpful, sometimes the wisdom of our compassionate mind can help us to understand what is capturing our attention in the first place. Without this understanding we can often end up avoiding, denying or ignoring something important that needs to be worked through. Let's look at an example.

Exercise: Bilal became aware that his mind was continually being pulled to a memory of feeling belittled, and treated badly, by his boss in front of other colleagues. When he completed his 'attention log' he found this was happening frequently, leaving him feeling a mixture of anger and shame. He tried to engage in mindfulness and soothing breathing, which did help a little in reducing the frequency and power of the experience. Bilal's therapist asked if he could access his compassionate self, and from this perspective, ask himself: 'What does your compassionate self understand about why your attention continues to be taken back to this memory?'

By engaging his compassionate self, with knowledge, understanding and wisdom, Bilal was able to recognise that his attention was getting brought back to this painful situation because he was cross that he hadn't stood up for himself. This made him want to address this, and with repeated practice in assertive behaviour over several weeks, Bilal was able to approach his boss and express his position, and sense of unfairness.

So, for Bilal it was helpful to learn that his compassionate mind was able to guide him to understanding there was an important 'function' (or reason) for why his attention was getting pulled towards a threat memory. Moreover, this awareness helped him recognise what he needed to do to support himself.

Let's spend some time practising compassionate attention together. To do this exercise, it might be helpful to first think about a recent situation in which your attention kept being pulled to a difficult issue or situation.

Exercise 2: What Sits Behind What We're Focusing On?

Sit in a comfortable and upright position. Spend a moment engaging in your soothing rhythm breathing (see pages 124–28). When you feel ready, bring to mind the qualities of your compassionate self – caring-commitment, strength and, in particular, wisdom. Then see if you can bring to mind a situation that has been preoccupying you. Be curious about what your mind might be searching for, trying to resolve, or work out. Guided by its wisdom, what does your compassionate mind think might sit behind this threat focus – for example, difficult threat emotions, concerns or fears you have, or a need of yours that has gone unmet? Why might your threat system be caught up with this situation, and what could this be telling you about how you feel or what you need? Make a few notes on this below.

_____

_____

_____

_____

If there is a particular reason why your attention is being caught up by your threat system, take a moment to reconnect again with your compassionate self. Given what you have learnt, what would your compassionate self suggest might be helpful for you?

What have you learnt from trying to bring a compassionate influence to your attention? Is there something helpful that you can do given this understanding?

_____

_____

_____

_____

As we discovered during our exploration of mindfulness in Chapter 8 (see pages 101–19), it can take a little time to practise bringing a compassionate attention and awareness to our lives. This is rarely easy to start with, but with time and practice, we can learn how to become more aware of our distress and begin to direct our attention in ways that will start to help us deal with our difficulties.

Chapter summary

In this chapter we have explored how our compassionate mind can guide our attention in ways that can be helpful.

What we have learnt together	My personal reflections on the chapter
1. It can be helpful to keep a log or diary to notice the nature and patterns of our attention on a daily basis. 2. Our attention is vulnerable to being hijacked by our threat system. 3. We can use mindfulness to bring our attention to the present moment, and thus redirect our attention away from threat-based, past or future-focused thinking. 4. We can use our compassionate minds to understand why our attention operates in particular ways, and redirect its focus in ways that are helpful.	

19 Putting our compassionate mind to work – Compassionate thinking

'A man's life is what his thoughts make it.'

– Marcus Aurelieus, Meditations, Book IV

We have many thoughts each day. In fact, some researchers have estimated that we have between *12,000 to 50,000* thoughts per day! Thoughts can have an infinite range of content. We can have positive, negative or neutral thoughts, thoughts that are compassionate, thoughts that are self-critical … We can have thoughts about the past, the future or what's going on now, and we can have profound thoughts and reflections, or thoughts that don't really make sense to us. One reality here though is that not all thoughts are made equal; in other words, different types of thoughts have a different impact upon us. It's likely that this makes intuitive sense. For example, bring to mind how you'd feel if you had positive thoughts about your performance in an interview or a competition, as opposed to thinking about yourself in a critical and hostile way. In this chapter we are going to explore how the way we think impacts upon the way we feel and behave, as well as how our thinking is, in itself, influenced by our emotion systems. We will also learn how we can bring greater balance to our thinking through our compassionate minds.

How much do we choose what we think?

If you consider the thoughts that you have in a day, do you choose them or do you become aware of them as they occur? Do you choose to have a negative thought about yourself, or do you just become aware of having a negative thought about yourself? Often, when we think this through, we can realise that so much of what goes on in our minds pops up without conscious control, awareness or desire. It is *created for us*, and *not by us*.

It might be that some aspects of how we think are influenced by what we've learnt in life. Let's look at Florence as an example here:

Example: Florence is forty-three years old, and has suffered with low mood throughout her life. Her father committed suicide when she was seven years old, and her mother, in her grief, struggled with depression throughout Florence's childhood. Her last memory of her father was of him telling her off for not tidying her room. She also recalled one time when her mother became very angry and shouted at Florence: 'It's all your fault your Dad died, he would still be here if you hadn't been such a difficult child!' Florence went on to believe that her father's death was her fault, and that the only way anyone would love her was if she was 'good', and behaved in a way that they wanted. When Florence was a teenager, her mother developed a drink problem, and when inebriated, would often say cruel things to her, such as 'You're useless, you don't do anything right' and 'You're such a let down'.

In therapy, Florence described various self-critical thoughts. Her inner self-critic often said things like 'You're useless', 'You can't do anything right' and 'You make mistakes and cause bad things to happen'. At first, Florence had no understanding of where these thoughts came from. In fact, she responded by saying 'I was born with something wrong with me. I'm a bad person.' It was only over time, with exploring her past experiences that Florence began to realise that she had learnt to think about herself in similar ways to how she had been talked to by others, in particular, by her mother. Through developing and using her compassionate mind, Florence was able to experience greater empathy for herself and for her struggle with self-criticism. She was able to see that the way she thought about herself was 'not her fault'.

We can see from the example above that Florence's early experiences had a significant impact on her life, and on the way in which she thought about herself. Most of us appreciate that, although we are born with the capacity to think in certain ways, we are not born thinking specific things about ourselves, or others. It may be that some of us are more analytical, pessimistic or liable to get caught up in worry than others. Some of us may be quite self-critical, whereas others are more self-compassionate. The ways in which we think about ourselves and others are shaped over time, through many routes, but one important way is through learning. The good news is that, just like many things that are learnt, we can also learn new ways (more compassionate ways) of thinking about ourselves, and practise these so that they become more accessible to us. We will return to this later.

Evolution has shaped the way we think

Although learning can shape the way we think about ourselves, we can look at an evolutionary understanding to make sense of why we can get caught up in certain patterns of thinking. In Chapter 1, we discussed the differences between our 'old brain' competencies that we share with other animals, and our 'new brain' competencies, such as imagination, planning, perspective taking, and so forth, linked to a more recently evolved part of our brain (see pages 3–15). We also saw how these same new brain abilities can be 'hijacked' by old brain emotions to create specific patterns of thinking, which in turn give rise to particular feelings (creating thinking-feeling vicious cycles), that can drive much of our distress. Our thoughts are naturally biased in a threat-focused way. This means that, when our threat system is activated, the nature and content of our thoughts tends to be related to old-brain threat feelings of anger, anxiety and shame. Here are some examples:

Threat emotion	Style of thinking	Content of thinking
Anxiety	Worry Danger-focused	'I've got to give a talk on Monday. I'll make mistakes and mess it all up.' 'The worst possible thing will happen.' 'The pain in my stomach is something serious – I think there's something seriously wrong with me, maybe it's cancer.'
Anger	Rumination Transgression/wrongness/unfairness-focused	'How dare she say that to me in the meeting! Who does she think she is? Why didn't I tell her what I thought of her?' Also, 'This is wrong'; 'This isn't fair.'
Shame	Self-criticism	'I can't do anything right – I'll always be a failure.' 'I'm a stupid, messed-up idiot.'

These are only examples, of course. We can also ruminate from an anxious or shame position (e.g. 'Why did I say that stupid thing at the meeting?'), and be future focused in our anger (e.g. thinking about revenge). Key here is that the content and process of our thinking is often shaped by the underlying threat emotion, which in turn may also stimulate more threat activation.

Better–safe–than–sorry thinking

As we explored in Chapter 3, our increased intelligence and cognitive abilities need to serve our most basic need – survival (see pages 23–8). It's no use having the brain power that can solve complex difficulties that we encounter in life if this same thinking also slowed down basic defensive behavioural responses (e.g. fight or flight) that help to keep us alive. Let's think of an example. Imagine taking a peaceful walk through a forest on a warm summer's day, and you step over a log. As you look down to the ground, you see an object on the floor that resembles like a snake. Without thinking, you immediately startle and jump away from it. Although this response might turn out to be unnecessary (i.e. it turns out it isn't actually a snake, only an old piece of rope), your mind cannot afford to take the chance to gamble with this. If, rather than jumping away, your more balanced thinking took over, this might cause you problems. For example, if you started thinking: 'That's strange, I've walked on this path hundreds of time, and never seen a snake' or 'I wonder if this is a poisonous snake, or one of those nice ones I've seen on TV that you can hold ...' your behavioural response would slow down, and you could be in big trouble if there was a snake. This threat-based, 'better-safe-than-sorry' way of thinking (and reacting) is automatic (i.e. you don't stop and think 'I'd better take this as a snake rather than a piece of rope') and designed by evolution to keep us safe. And over billions of years it has been species that were able to respond in this self-protective way to dangerous environments and situations that were more likely to survive and pass on their genes. The take-home message is that, when in threat conditions, we tend to think in quick, automatic and non-rational ways that facilitate our survival. But (and this is a *big* but), we can end up paying a price for this better-safe-than-sorry thinking. In modern-day contexts, where survival threats might be less pervasive, our minds continue to operate in the same way with thoughts that might be illogical, unrealistic and ultimately unhelpful. Here are three common better-safe-than-sorry thinking patterns:

- *Jumping to conclusions* – quickly forming an opinion in the absence of sufficient evidence. Tending to think that negative things will happen (e.g. 'Because she didn't say hello to me, that means she doesn't like me').

- *Overgeneralising* – one bad experience (e.g. a job interview failure) extends to all similar situations in the future (e.g. 'I will fail at all future job interviews').

- *Dichotomous thinking* – seeing things as all 'good' or all 'bad', otherwise referred to as *black-and-white thinking*.

Self-reflection: Can you think of a time when you found yourself thinking in any of these 'better-safe-than sorry' ways? What did you think about yourself and the situation? If you were thinking about another person, what assumptions did you make about them?

_____

_____

_____

The fact that this happens, that our thinking minds become biased in such a way, is not our fault. Rather, it results from evolutionary processes that prioritise ancient (old brain), rapid, protective responses around safety. These in turn influence how our new brain 'thinking' operates (see Chapter 1, page 12, for a reminder of how our old brain can shape our new brain). When we feel threatened in some way, our thinking will also become shaped and biased in a threat-focused way as well. Having compassionate wisdom means that we can understand and appreciate this truth of life. In turn having this insight will then help us to learn ways to mindfully and compassionately work with this truth and the problems it poses.

Using our compassionate minds to engage our threat-system-based thinking

There are a number of ways that we can work with threat-based thinking, and we will explore these below. Let's look at this in more detail by following a series of steps.

Step 1: Learning to notice threat-system-based thoughts, and our reactions to them

We can learn to notice the types of threat-based thoughts we have, the content of these, and the way we typically deal with them when they arise. This can be useful as being aware of such thoughts may provide the opportunity of a 'gap' between automatically following them – we can pause and remind ourselves that thoughts are not necessarily facts. It may give space for us to choose whether it would be helpful to follow what our mind is telling us, or whether we need to focus on different, and potentially more helpful, thoughts. To support you in this process we have created Worksheet 19.1 below. If you're willing, spend a day paying attention to and recording the content and nature of your threat system based thoughts.

Worksheet 19.1: Threat-system-based thought monitoring form

Time of day	Type of thought (e.g. threat-based - worrying, ruminating, or reassuring)	Content of thought (e.g. about work, family, health, the future)	How did this thought affect my feelings? (e.g. anxious, angry, sad, happy)	How did I deal with the thought? (e.g. ignored it, tried to stop it, tried to push it out of mind, acted on it)
Morning				
Afternoon				
Evening				

Self-reflection: What did you learn about your thoughts from this exercise? Did you notice any patterns in your thinking?

_____

_____

_____

_____

Sometimes completing this form can be useful in itself. Becoming aware of what is happening in our minds, the reactions we have to our own thoughts, and how these may exacerbate some of our difficulties can motivate us to think about things in a different way. This may help to provide an awareness from which we learn to relate (or respond) to our thoughts in a more helpful manner. For example, when Jess completed this form, she noticed that she spent a lot of time (and quite a bit of energy) in the day trying not to think about her unhappiness in her current relationship – trying to push these thoughts out of her mind, or finding distractions so that she wouldn't have to focus on them. In contrast, Pete found that he responded to his worries about financial problems by thinking over and over about how the problems came about in quite an obsessive and ruminatory manner. Both Jess and Pete recognised that although understandable, their attempts to manage their threat-based thoughts were actually quite tiring, and didn't seem to make much difference in preventing them.

Self-reflection: Spend some time considering the way that you cope with your own thoughts. Are your attempts helpful? Are there any unintended consequences?

_____

_____

_____

If you do find that your current ways of trying to cope with your thoughts are unhelpful, the following exercise might help.

Exercise 1 – Mindfulness of Thoughts

Over the coming day, try to notice your thoughts as they arise in your mind, as you did with the thought monitoring form (Worksheet 19.1 above). In particular, notice when you become overly connected to, or preoccupied with, certain types of thoughts, particularly those that are threat-based (e.g. worry, rumination, and self-criticism). When you become aware of these, gently, and without judgement, bring your attention back to a neutral anchor, such as your breathing or the sounds around you. If you notice that your mind is trying to push them out, ignore them, fight with them, control or criticise them (or yourself for having them), see if you can just notice this, and then gently bring your attention back to focusing upon your breath, or the sounds around you.

As best you can, continue with this way of neutrally observing and not engaging with your thoughts, regardless of your mind's pull to fight, avoid or control them. If it helps to remind yourself, take a look back to Chapter 8 (pages 101–19) where we explore mindfulness in more detail.

Self-reflection: What was it like paying attention to your thoughts in this way? How did you find trying to respond to them mindfully?

_____

_____

_____

Step 2: Bringing greater balance to our thinking

Whilst learning to notice our thoughts, and using mindfulness as a way to ground and anchor ourselves in the 'here and now' can be very helpful, we may also need to work with the content of our thoughts in a more direct way. Although it's not our fault that our thinking can become threat-focused, it may be helpful to use our compassionate minds to create more balanced and helpful ways of thinking. To begin with, let's explore the differences between threat-based thinking and compassionate thinking:

	Threat-based thinking	Compassionate thinking
Focus	Narrowly tied to the cause, or trigger of the threat	Open and broad We are able to see the 'wood for the trees'
Form	Repetitive, ruminative, and lacking flexibility	Flexible and balanced We can notice, but not over-identify with, the thought
Content	Non-rational, negative – 'better safe than sorry'	Underpinned by care, support, warmth and compassion - balanced
Intent	Guided by nature of threat and specific threat emotion, e.g. • Intent to punish or seek revenge, if based on anger • Intent to avoid or appease, if based on anxiety	Validates, empathises and supports Intention to be sensitive and helpful

The purpose of developing compassionate ways of thinking is not to create 'positive' thoughts – although sometimes people do develop these. Rather, the aim is to train our minds to think in sensitive and helpful ways. We do this by trying to generate a broader, more balanced perspective to our thinking. We root our thinking into our intention to alleviate our and other people's suffering. This is not simply a process of thinking in a logical and rational way, it is important to connect with (if we can) an emotional, heartfelt feeling of care and warmth alongside our rationality. To help with this, we are again going to engage the part of us that is able to 'do the work' – our compassionate mind. In this next section we are going to introduce you to thought records, which can help us attend to, slow down and refocus our busy mind, and generate a balanced view of difficult situations.

Exercise 2: Compassionate Thought Form

In this exercise we will look at how we can use our compassionate minds to support us in times of suffering, where our new brain capacity for thinking, reasoning and imagination may be contributing to or compounding our distress. We're going to explore this by using Joe's example of losing his job. We then encourage you to have a go at completing Worksheet 19.1.

Example: Joe is a 45-year-old married man with two children. He has worked in the same factory for fifteen years, doing long shifts, but his pay barely covered the bills. Unfortunately Joe was recently made redundant, and when he came to therapy, reported that he had been feeling depressed and anxious for the past two months.

There are three steps to working with this form.

Step 1 – Exploring our thoughts and feelings after a recent difficulty

The first step involves columns 1 to 3, in which you bring to mind a recent situation that you found difficult, and consider the types of threat-based thoughts you had, and how these left you feeling. Let's look at how Joe got on with this.

	Column 1 **Triggering Events**	Column 2 **Unhelpful or Upsetting Thoughts and Images**	Column 3 **Feelings and Emotions**
	What actually happened? What was the trigger?	What went through my mind? What am I thinking about others and their thoughts about me? What am I thinking about myself and my future?	What are my main feelings and emotions?
Joe's answer:	*'I was called into the boss's office and told that I was being made redundant.'*	*'I am not good enough. What will my family say? My brother will be critical – he always is. I will not be able to support my family. We may lose the house. No one will employ me at my age. People will judge and criticise me, thinking I have done something wrong.'*	*'I feel sad, ashamed and angry.'*

So now that we've had a look at Joe's answers, take some time to think about a recent situation that you can base your thought record on, and then make some notes for columns 1, 2 and 3. There is space for your answers in Worksheet 19.2 on page 245.

Step 2 – Bringing balance to our minds

The second step involves completing column 4, 'Thought balancing'. Before you have a go at this, it is crucial that you spend some time connecting with the part of you that can look at this situation in a different, more balanced, sensitive and helpful way. As you can probably guess, this means getting in touch with your compassionate mind. See if you can spend some time engaging in this, initially connecting with your soothing breathing first, and then linking in with the qualities of your compassionate self – caring-commitment, wisdom and strength. If it helps, spend some time doing one of the experiences that we explored in Chapters 12, 13 or 14.

You will also notice that there are different subheadings (empathy and validation for your distress, compassionate attention, compassionate thinking and compassionate behaviour) in column 4. Let's have a look at the subheadings (taking one at a time), then take a look at the questions in column 4 and Joe's answers to those questions.

Empathy and validation for your distress

It can be important to start with validating and having empathy for where you are – for the distress you've been experiencing. For example, 'It is understandable I feel like this because I have been living with this for so long now. My threat system gets activated as soon as I start thinking about these struggles and this is not my fault.'

> Joe's answer: 'It's understandable that I've been thinking and feeling like this. Losing a job is very distressing, and it's natural to sometimes worry about the future. This is not my fault.'

Compassionate attention

Similar to what we explored in Chapter 18, it can be helpful to notice where your attention is being pulled into (most often the threat system, and in a narrow focused way). In comparison, consider what might be more helpful to pay attention to. This could be noticing and stepping back from negative 'loops in the mind', or trying to focus on something that provides a broader and more helpful context (e.g. by paying attention to occasions when things have been different / when things went well).

> Joe's answer: 'It is helpful for me to remember that I have also had successes at work, and worked very hard and with good feedback from colleagues and managers.'

Compassionate thinking

Here, rather than being critical and ruminating about thoughts, we are trying to find ways to bring an alternative, helpful, supportive and balanced perspective to the situation we are struggling with. It may help to think about what you would say to a friend in the same situation, or to think about what somebody who cares for you would say to you, if they were aware of your thoughts. Box 19.1 below lists some examples of compassionate thoughts.

Box 19.1: Examples of compassionate thoughts/statements

- It is understandable that I feel like this at the moment
- Life is hard and other people experience situations like this
- I could spend some time thinking about the struggles I have managed in the past
- My automatic 'better safe than sorry' threat-detection system has been activated, so I'm likely to think in a biased way. This is understandable and not my fault

- This is a moment of pain/sorrow/suffering, is a natural part of life, but it will pass
- These thoughts are just events in my mind, rather than reflections about me
- Just because this is hard it doesn't mean that things will always be hard
- Perhaps I can look at the bigger picture – is there anything I'm missing, or minimising because my mind is only focusing on negative experiences?

Joe's answer: 'Being made redundant was not specifically about me – my colleagues also lost their jobs. It's not my fault – I worked hard, and had a good review last month. The financial situation has caused this. Friends and family have been supportive – they know the reality of the situation and that this wasn't due to anything I've done wrong. This is not an indication of my worth as a human being.'

Compassionate behaviour

Holding in mind the difficulty, think about how your compassionate self can help you to take action, and change your behaviour. For example, if you are avoiding a situation or finding something difficult to do, how can your compassionate self help you? Can you ask for support from someone you feel safe with, so that you can move in a direction that will help you to alleviate some of your difficulties? We will explore compassionate behaviour in more detail in the Chapter 21.

Joe's answers: 'Although it is hard, I will speak to some friends about how I'm feeling. I'll also speak to my family – it's OK to show my feelings rather than bottling them up. On Monday I'm going to go to the Jobcentre to see what else is out there.'

Step 3 – Noticing any changes

Engage your soothing breathing and compassionate self and spend some time reading over what you've put down in column 4 with a warm supportive voice tone. Notice and write down in column 5 how you feel now about this situation.

Joe's answer: 'I still feel sad about losing my job – and a bit angry, but I'm not blaming or criticising myself. I feel less stressed about it all.'

You can find Joe's full, completed thought form in Box 19.2. Once you feel familiar with the process, have a go at completing your own thought form (Worksheet 19.2). Box 19.3 on page 246 lists some of the common difficulties with thought records, and offers some helpful hints to guide you in completing your own form.

Box 19.2 Joe's Completed Compassionate Thought Record

Column 1 Triggering events	Column 2 Unhelpful or upsetting thoughts and images	Column 3 Feelings and emotions	Column 4 Thought balancing – 'helpful' or 'balanced' thoughts	Column 5 Understanding and change in feelings
What actually happened? What was the trigger?	*What am I thinking about others and their thoughts about me? What am I thinking about myself?*	*What are my main feelings and emotions?*	*What would I say to a friend?* *What compassionate alternatives might there be?*	*Write down any change in your feelings*
'I was called in to the boss's office and told that I was being made redundant.'	'I am not good enough.' 'What will my family say? My brother will be critical, he always is.' 'I will not be able to support my family, we may lose the house.' 'No one will employ me at my age.' 'People will judge and criticise me, thinking I have done something wrong.'	'I feel sad, ashamed and angry.'	**Empathy for my distress** 'It's understandable that I've been thinking and feeling like this. Losing a job is very distressing, and it's natural to sometimes worry about the future. This is not my fault.' **Compassionate attention** 'It is helpful for me to remember that I have also had successes at work, and worked very hard and with good feedback from colleagues and managers.' **Compassionate thinking** 'Being made redundant was not personal to me – my colleagues also lost their jobs.' 'It's not my fault – I worked hard, and had a good review last month. The financial situation has caused this.' 'Friends and family have been supportive – they know the reality of the situation and that this wasn't due to anything I've done wrong. This is not an indication of my worth as a human being.' **Compassionate behaviour** 'Although it is hard, I will speak to some friends about how I'm feeling. I'll also speak to my family – it's OK to show my feelings rather than bottle them up. On Monday I'm going to go to the Jobcentre to see what else is out there.'	'I still feel sad about losing my job – and a bit angry, but I am not blaming or criticising myself.' 'I am a good worker and will get through this.'

Worksheet 19.2: Compassionate Thought Record

Column 1 Triggering Events	Column 2 Unhelpful or Upsetting Thoughts and Images	Column 3 Feelings and Emotions	Column 4 Thought balancing – 'Helpful' or 'Balanced' Thoughts	Column 5 Understanding and Change in Feelings
What actually happened? What was the trigger?	*What am I thinking about others and their thoughts about me? What am I thinking about myself?*	*What are my main feelings and emotions?*	*What would I say to a friend? What compassionate alternatives might there be?*	*Write down any change in your feelings*
			Empathy for my distress	
			Compassionate attention	
			Compassionate thinking	
			Compassionate behaviour	

Self-reflection: How did you find this exercise? What was it like to bring a compassionate perspective to your difficulties?

_____

_____

_____

Box 19.3: Common difficulties and helpful hints for thought forms

Common difficulties	Helpful hints
I try to focus on my thoughts but then get stuck in 'What ifs'. I'll never get better at this.	This is a common difficulty. It's helpful here to remind yourself that your threat system has just been triggered, and that it's understandable to struggle with this.
	Try not to be disheartened. See if you can gently return to soothing rhythm breathing (see pages 123–28) and focus on your compassionate self – with its wisdom, strength and caring-commitment. Perhaps use your safe place or compassionate team and remind yourself that learning a new skill takes time. Notice the thoughts and remind yourself that thoughts are not facts and they always evolve and change.
	Ask yourself, what you would say to a friend in this scenario – would you be so hard on your friend?
I set time aside to write in my thought record, but couldn't think of any thoughts to write about.	That's OK. Sometimes the best time to write thought records is when you notice your

	emotions change. For example, if you notice that you feel sad, or angry, or anxious.
I lose concentration and start thinking 'I have lots of other stuff I should be doing'.	Our minds are always thinking about what we did in the past, or what we should be doing in the future. This is normal. Once again, engage your soothing breathing. See if you can tap back in to your compassionate motivation to remind yourself why it's important to spend time working on your thinking (it may be helpful to look back at Section IV pages 163–6, to remind yourself about this). Perhaps ask yourself, using your compassionate mind, 'Is this other stuff more important to me?' If so, can you find time to do both?

Compassionate flash cards

Although compassionate thought forms can be very helpful, especially as a way of training our 'thinking', they might be tricky to carry around and therefore not very accessible when we might most benefit from using them. Instead, it can be helpful to develop ways in which we can address our thinking in the here and now. One such accessible measure is to use compassionate flash cards. These are small cards that help you to focus on a particular issue and can help you to engage your compassionate self, you at your best, or connect with your ideal compassionate other. The flash cards can hold key messages, pictures or phrases that can be supportive and encouraging. They can encourage you to practise, and they can remind you of what your compassionate self would say or how he/she would react and think in particular situations. The flash card may just act as a reminder of your commitment to becoming your compassionate self. They can be pocket- or wallet-size, which can be left next to your bed, on your fridge, or next to your mirror.

Technology has improved quite a lot since we started using flash cards! You may prefer to leave or send messages on your phone, or use an app. Many of our clients also use pictures that remind them of a key helpful message, thought or experience.

Chapter summary

In this chapter we've learnt that whilst our thinking can easily be hijacked by our threat system, by engaging our compassionate minds this can help us to bring a more balanced and helpful perspective to situations.

What we have learnt together	My personal reflections on the chapter
1. We can train our minds to become aware of their present content and functioning, and to stand back and observe the patterns of our thoughts and emotions with compassion.	
2. When our emotions are in control we tend to jump to conclusions, overgeneralise or make global assumptions about how awful future events will be.	
3. Compassionate thought records can help to bring a different, more balanced perspective to difficult situations.	

20 Putting our compassionate mind to work – Compassionate engagement of emotion

'Out of your vulnerabilities will come your strength.'

– *Sigmund Freud*

In this chapter we are going to explore how we can use our compassionate mind to work with difficult emotions. Emotions add texture to our experiences in life; they add colour and depth, richness and interest. Without emotion, so much of our life would be hollow – stripped of meaning, energy and motivation. However, emotions can also be painful and difficult, and are often unwanted. We can spend much of our time trying to fight or avoid experiencing certain feelings and emotions. Unfortunately, this way of trying to manage them can create more pain and distress. In fact, much of our work as therapists is helping people to find ways to understand and better manage their emotions, and the pain they cause – whether that's the overwhelming fear that comes with social anxiety or agoraphobia; the difficulties with anger or shame that come with many depressions and traumas; or the struggle with sadness and grief that accompany bereavements, separations or endings in relationships.

In this chapter we're going to explore some of the emotions we commonly struggle with. We'll explore reasons for why this might be, and crucially, how compassion can help us to feel more at ease in tolerating, experiencing and expressing our emotions in adaptive ways.

Bringing your compassionate mind to work with your emotions

How we understand and deal with our emotions partly depends on the different factors that have shaped them over time. These include differences in our genes, life experiences, temperament and personality, and our current relationships and environments. Crucially, the way we relate to or manage our emotions can vary in many ways. Psychologists suggest there are some key aspects to what might be considered to be healthy, helpful or adaptive management of emotions. These include:

- Detecting an emotion once it has been triggered

- Describing and putting words to the emotion experienced

- Understanding and making sense of why we are feeling what we are feeling

- Tolerating and using the emotion we are feeling in a way that is helpful.

These skills are sometimes referred to as *emotion regulation* – a term used by psychologists and therapists to refer to our attempts and ability to manage our emotions in helpful and healthy ways. Having adaptive emotion regulation skills means being able to notice, describe, experience, tolerate and express emotions in a useful or positive way. Conversely, poor emotion regulation skills involve a compromised ability to understand, tolerate and express emotions. In this chapter, we are going to spend some time seeing how our compassionate mind can help us to become more sensitive, understanding and competent in the way we experience and use our emotions. In other words, we are going to see how your compassionate self can help you cultivate your emotion regulation skills. We will explore this in a number of steps:

Step 1: Noticing and identifying emotions

Similar to the insights we explored in Chapters 18 and 19, paying attention to our experiences in a mindful way can play an important role in us being able to manage these in a helpful and wise manner. It is similar with our emotions. If we're unaware, or *unmindful*, that an emotion has been triggered inside us, there is a risk that this emotion plays through us. In other words, it plays its tune, which may be a tune that is fitting for the situation, but equally, the tune it plays may not be so meaningful for the situation. For example, if we are not aware that anger has been triggered in us, we may be in an important meeting and begin to behave in an aggressive, critical and blaming way to our boss or colleagues, without realising that this is happening or what has caused it to happen.

One way that we can learn to notice our emotions is by paying attention to how they feel in the body. Often we don't just experience one discrete emotion at a given time but a mixture of different emotions, and we can shift between emotional responses in a fluid way. For example, if you were starting a new job, you might experience a variety of emotions – you might feel excited, but you may also feel anxious and slightly nervous. In the case of an argument, you may feel angry, as well as anxious and/or upset. Each of these emotions comes with a set of information (or signals) about what to do in that situation. In other words, emotions can give us information about what is important, threatening, valued and fair to us, and can direct us to act in a way that is consistent with this underlying need or experience. For example, we often feel anxiety as tightness in our stomach, shakiness in our legs, sweaty hands, tension in our neck and shoulders, and/or dryness in our mouth. These physiological responses can urge our body to move away from a threat, real or perceived, in order to be safe. When angry, we often feel a tension in our jaw, shoulders, arms and hands. This signals our readiness to fight for something that is important to us, our values and our goals, or against something that has threatened us.

Noticing how emotions feel in our body can help us understand what that feeling is urging us to do. Having this awareness can help us to know and decide whether this urged action would be helpful, appropriate and useful. Noticing our feelings can also guide us towards a helpful way of expressing, communicating and managing that emotion. For example, if you notice feeling angry and having the urge to punch the wall, this could be quite helpful – to both the wall and your hand! Conversely, diminished or absent awareness of how our emotions 'show up' in our body and what they are urging us to do might inhibit this process of reflection and adaptive emotional management, and instead lead to automatically reacting on emotion in ways that might be unhelpful. So, lacking awareness that we are angry and feeling the urge to punch the wall is more likely to lead to a damaged wall and certainly, a damaged hand. The first step, therefore, towards 'healthy' emotion regulation is to learn how to tune into, or listen to our feelings and physical reactions, mindfully noticing them and the way they feel in our bodies. Let's start by trying out the exercise in Worksheet 20.1, below:

Worksheet 20.1: Recognising how our emotions show themselves in the body

Emotion	What was happening when I experienced this emotion? What triggered the emotion?	Where did I notice this feeling in my body?	What did my body want to do when I felt like this?
Anger			
Anxiety			
Sadness			
Disgust			
Shame			
Guilt			
Pride			
Joy			
Contentment			

Self-reflection: What did you learn about your emotions from this exercise? Was it easier to notice how some emotions were triggered than others? Was it easier to recall and notice some emotions than others?

_____

_____

_____

_____

Try not to worry if you found identifying certain – or even most – of the emotions on the above worksheet difficult. Lots of people also find it hard to do this, and there can be many reasons why this is the case. It can be helpful over time to come back to this Worksheet 20.1 and see if you find differences in your awareness of these emotions.

We can also look at monitoring and learning about our emotions in a different way. Rather than thinking backwards in time, it can be helpful to spend some time looking out for, noticing and tracking our emotions as they emerge during the day. This helps us to become more aware of our feelings, and have a better sense of how the emotion 'shows up' in our body. Remember, emotions often come with a physiological 'pattern' to them, and the more that we can recognise our emotions when we experience them, the better chance we have to regulate and use them in a helpful way, rather than them leading us. Let's try this by monitoring our emotions on Worksheet 20.2.

Worksheet 20.2: Emotion Monitoring Form

Time of day	What situation am I in, and who am I with?	What emotion do I feel?	Where do I feel it in my body?	What does my body want to do?
Morning				
Afternoon				
Evening				

Self-reflection: What did you learn from monitoring your emotions for a day? Did certain emotions show up more often than others?

_____

_____

_____

It's helpful sometimes to continue monitoring our emotions over a longer period – for example, a week or two. This can give us a better sense of which emotions we experience more frequently, and highlight those we rarely experience, or that are absent or blocked. Although it's easy to focus just on the emotions we experience regularly, it can also be useful to notice – and then try to understand why – we may not experience certain emotions regularly. For example, although it might seem like a good thing if we don't experience much anger in life, it depends on what situations we've been in. If we've not experienced anger because the situation did not call for, or require an angry response, that's fine. However, let's imagine that you are treated in a very disrespectful or demeaning way by a shop assistant or colleague. It might be that without access to anger, it's much harder to stick up for yourself, challenge and be assertive in a helpful way.

Noticing and monitoring our emotional reactions (as in the example of Worksheet 20.2, above) can also enrich our understanding of how certain emotions affect us over time. For example, a short-term experience of anger may enable us to challenge someone who has treated us unfairly, or blocked us from achieving something that's important to us. In the moment this happens, anger may help us to mobilise energy, direct attention and instigate a behavioural response (e.g. assertively confronting the person), which can bring us closer to our goals, or prevent further unfair treatment. However, if we continue to experience anger after the incident has passed, this may become problematic. For example, we may be in a situation where there is no real threat, transgression, or block to our goals, but by continuing to feel angry, we might react in an anger-driven way (e.g. confrontationally or even aggressively), rather than in a neutral, balanced and helpful way.

Step 2: Making sense of our emotions

Whilst we may learn to notice and identify emotions as they arise, a significant difficulty for many people involves *understanding why they are feeling the way they are*. One client told us: 'I can tell you that I'm feeling angry. I can notice the feeling in my body, but I can't tell you for the life of me why I am feeling like this.' Other people may *invalidate* their emotions. Invalidation here means that we see our emotions as something not valid, and discredit them, feeling they are somehow incorrect, non-understandable, or even wrong. Another client said, 'I shouldn't be feeling sad, I shouldn't be crying – nothing that bad has happened for me to feel like this.' Unfortunately, when we invalidate our feelings, we often create a threat response. It is as if someone is standing next to us and shouting at us, 'You shouldn't be feeling like this, there's something wrong with you!'

How might we learn to validate and understand our emotions? Well, when we notice that we are invalidating our emotions, it could be helpful to start with validating the invalidation – that is, to try and see how it might be understandable that we invalidate our emotions based on what we know about our previous experiences (for example, being raised in a house in which we are taught that emotions are bad or wrong in some way can teach us to do the same). Having wisdom in this instance means:

• Recognising and understanding the cause of your suffering

• Knowing that we have no choice over the design of our body and brain or the life that we have been born into

• Knowing that experiencing and working through painful feelings can be difficult.

Let's look at an example:

> *Example:* Jake was raised in a family where he learnt that sadness was not an acceptable emotion to feel. His parents provided for him and he had a good education, but whenever he expressed sadness (for example, if he was upset about something going on at school), his parents would shout at him, and say, 'What's wrong with you? Stop being such a baby girl and toughen up!' Through his childhood and adolescence, Jake learned to suppress feelings of sadness and distress. Although a successful businessman now, he came to therapy feeling low in mood and 'detached' following the death of his best friend from cancer. He was able to voice that he felt very sad about losing his friend, but quickly added, 'I shouldn't feel like this, he died ages ago. I should be strong and get on with things – it's pathetic I'm struggling like this.' With the help of therapy, Jake was able to develop his compassionate

self, and through this he came to see that it was understandable, given his upbringing, that he struggled to experience sadness, and why he had developed a very invalidating stance with regards to some of his emotional experiences. Although difficult, over time he was able to see that it was OK to feel sad about losing his best friend, that he was experiencing a natural response to the death of someone he loved very much.

Self-reflection: Now, let's try to apply this to your experiences. Consider a time when you experienced a difficult emotion, or identify an emotion you're struggling with at the moment. Take a few minutes to think about this. It might help to start by connecting with your soothing breathing and compassionate self. From this part of you, look at the emotion you are experiencing and consider how you might validate it, seeing it as an understandable experience, given what you know about emotions in general, and yourself. If you find it difficult to validate your experience, consider how you might do this if a friend was struggling with a similar experience and you wanted to help them to see this as understandable. How would you try and validate their experience, and the way they are feeling? How might you empathise with, or understand why they are feeling the way they do? If it's helpful, make a few notes below:

_____

_____

_____

_____

What was it like to try to validate your feelings?

_____

_____

Were there any obstacles to you doing this? If so, what were they? How could your compassionate self help you with this?

_____

_____

Step 3: Using your compassionate mind to help tolerate your emotions

Some people are able to engage in the first two steps above – noticing and understanding their emotions. However, what gets in the way of helpfully managing their emotions is the fear associated with truly connecting with them. For many, this is linked to the fear that if they feel a difficult emotion, this will overwhelm them in some way.

Example: Ruth came to therapy able to notice difficult emotions (in her case, anger), and was able to bring wisdom to and validate why she was feeling the way she was. She recalled that as a child, her mother used to become very angry when her father was late home from work. In these angry moments, her mother would shout, swear and say some cruel things about Ruth and her brother, and would often stop speaking to them for a few days afterwards.

Whilst Ruth recognised that it was understandable that she found experiencing anger difficult, she also feared that if she allowed herself to feel angry, she might 'end up like Mum was'. So to protect herself – and the people she loved – she worked hard to suppress her anger, and would use various strategies to ensure she didn't become angry (e.g. drinking, avoiding people who made her angry, or trying hard to come across as a 'non-angry person'). Unfortunately, avoiding experiencing and expressing her anger meant that other people often found her either distant or cold. Moreover, her alcohol consumption in itself began to lead to problems.

In therapy Ruth learned many of the skills we explored in Sections III and IV, and with support from her compassionate self began to find ways of experiencing (and tolerating) her anger without needing to shut it down, avoid, or suppress it. In particular, she found it helpful to connect with her breathing rhythm, body posture and imagine the strength of the compassionate self as a way of doing this. Over time, this became a little easier, and gradually Ruth learned to express her anger in a way that was helpful and safe.

Self-reflection: Take a moment to think about an emotion that you find difficult to tolerate, or feel. As a clue, think about emotions you try to avoid feeling, or try to control or block in some way. It might help to think of a recent situation when you found it difficult to experience a particular emotion. Once you've identified an emotion, spend some time working through the following experiential exercise:

Exercise 1: Tolerating Difficult Emotions

Sit in an upright but comfortable position. Engage in your soothing rhythm breathing and friendly facial expression (see pages 122–28). Allow your breathing to slow a little, and gently rest your attention in the flow of breathing in, and breathing out. Stay with this for sixty seconds, or so.

Now, like an actor getting in a role, bring to mind your compassionate self. Spend some time connecting with its qualities – commitment, wisdom and in particular, your strength and courage. Notice your body posture, voice tone and facial expression. If it helps, return to Chapter 12 to connect with this practice more fully.

When you feel ready, bring to mind the emotion that you find difficult to experience, or tolerate. Maybe you can hold in mind the situation that last triggered it.

How would your compassionate self – this strong, wise and committed part of you – help you to tolerate this difficult emotion? What might they say, do or suggest that would help you with this?

If you feel yourself getting overwhelmed by the threat emotion, reconnect with your breathing and embodiment of your compassionate self. When you feel ready, bring yourself back to connect with the emotion you feel fearful of. Allow yourself to be in the presence of this feeling from a perspective of security, groundedness and courage that your compassionate self gives you. Notice what happens to the intensity of the fear or concerns you may have around experiencing this emotion.

Try imagining that in front of you is the 'you' who is struggling to manage this difficult emotion. As your compassionate self, with its strength, wisdom and commitment, imagine approaching this struggling version of you. What would you want to say or do to help? How could you support this part of you to tolerate this difficult feeling? Perhaps you could offer some words of care, understanding, reassurance, and encouragement?

When you feel ready, finish the exercise and make a few notes about your experience below.

Self-reflection: What was this exercise like? How did it feel to approach the difficult emotion from the perspective of your compassionate self?

_____

_____

_____

Was there anything that prevented your compassionate self from helping with this difficult emotion? If so, what might your compassionate self need to help with this (e.g. a greater sense of strength and groundedness)?

_____

_____

Looking to the future, how can your compassionate self help you to approach and manage this difficult emotion?

_____

_____

Step 4: Learning to express your emotions

As we explored in Chapter 3, emotions evolved to offer adaptive functions within particular environmental contexts; for example, sadness can signal the need for support and connection, often following an experience of loss or separation. Disgust is linked to the need to expel or get away from something that is noxious, or perceived to be unpleasant. Anxiety evolved to move us away from things that are threatening, whereas anger can stimulate our ability to challenge and be assertive when there has been a transgression. However, while these evolved functions make sense, expressing emotions can be very difficult for many of us. Sometimes this can be because we have never been taught how to express our feelings. For example, if our carers found it difficult to express their emotions, or failed to teach us how to express emotions in a helpful and healthy way, it's understandable that we may struggle with this later in life. For others, there can be fears associated with expressing certain emotions, as it was for Ruth, who feared that experiencing and expressing her anger would turn her into a hurtful person, like her mum.

In other words, expressing certain emotions can stimulate our threat systems, and make us feel vulnerable to other people's responses (e.g. their anger, anxiety, disgust) and behaviour (e.g. we might fear that they will reject, leave or punish us). We can also form threat-based judgements about ourselves (e.g. 'What sort of person would get anxious at something so small?'). When our threat system is activated in the face of a difficult emotion, it is trying to keep us safe by telling us, 'Don't say anything – keep it to yourself, or else …'. Of course in this case our threat system is doing its job, trying to protect us from physical or emotional pain. However, blocking or suppressing our emotions or expressions in this way can lead to unintended consequences, such as other people failing to recognise our needs, or walking all over us. For others, suppressing emotions can lead to a sense of 'emotional hoarding', which may ultimately lead to an emotional eruption. Let's reflect in more detail about how this works for you.

Self-reflection: Think about the emotion you find most difficult to express to others. Which emotion(s) is this, and what is your fear about expressing this emotion?

_____

_____

_____

How do you usually deal with this fear/concern (e.g. keep things to yourself, avoid this emotion, hide, block or numb it?)

_____

_____

_____

_____

Are there any unintended consequences of your safety strategies – of not expressing your emotions?

_____

_____

_____

One of the key difficulties in expressing emotions is learning to manage our fears and concerns about doing so. It can be helpful to bring your compassionate mind to help with this struggle.

Exercise 2: How Can Your Compassionate Mind Help You With Expressing Your Emotions?

Take a moment to connect with your soothing rhythm breathing (see pages 124–28). When you feel ready, bring to mind the qualities of your compassionate self, or your ideal compassionate other. Try your best to connect with a sense of caring-motivation, wisdom and strength. When you feel ready, from the compassionate part of you, look back at your understanding of your struggle to tolerate an emotion (Step 3). What does your compassionate self recognise about this? What would it want to say about this fear or concern? Can it see that it is understandable in some way? Take sixty seconds or so to reflect on this. Make some notes if that's helpful.

Given its understanding about this difficulty, what would your compassionate self like to do to help you with this struggle – to help you to express this emotion in a helpful and 'wise' way? How might the compassionate self help you to take steps towards expressing this emotion, when appropriate? How would your compassionate self encourage you to express or manage this emotion? Consider some of the following ideas:

* Would it be helpful to tell someone how you feel?

* Would it be helpful to let someone know how their behaviour left you feeling?

* Would it be helpful to write about how you feel?

* Could you talk to a friend who is not involved in this situation, and get their support and ideas about how to do this?

Self-reflection: How did you find that exercise? Could you imagine how your compassionate self could help you with this?

_____

_____

_____

_____

_____

_____

Often, people find that pulling together some of the central aspects of their compassionate selves facilitates the ability to express their emotions. For example, it takes the wisdom to know that, although understandable and unintended, the non-expression of emotions (or the acting out on emotions!), is causing distress for ourselves, and sometimes, for others. It takes a commitment to care to be sensitive to how painful emotions can be, and to work towards alleviating some of this pain. And it is through connecting with compassionate courage and strength that empowers us to tolerate, and express our emotions in a helpful way, as well as confront our fears about them. Box 20.1 below lists some tips for expressing emotions, which you may find helpful.

Box 20.1: Tips for expressing emotions

Tips – expressing emotions

It can be helpful to practise expressing your emotions and feelings in different ways. For example, you might:

- Write down on a piece of paper the emotion you're struggling to express, and how you would like to express this to someone else if you could

- Practise expressing your emotions and feelings out loud – maybe you could even try saying these in front of a mirror or if it feels safer, use your imagination to picture expressing this emotion in a helpful way

- Rehearse expressing your emotions with someone (a friend or family member) that you feel safe with

- Notice how others might express their emotions, and see if you can learn anything about healthy and helpful expression, i.e. how are they choosing their words, what is their voice tone, posture, eye gaze, facial expression, etc.

With continued practice, you will gradually find it easier to express some of the emotions you previously avoided, bottled up, or, conversely, lost yourself to, or acted out. As with any change, you may experience some difficulty with this initially. This would be particularly the case if you have expectations that in expressing emotion, everything will be straightforward, that others will listen and accept them, and that you will feel better. In our experience, this isn't always the case, and sometimes this is because other people (those who see or receive the expressed emotion) do not know how to deal with this change in behaviour. Being compassionate here would involve recognising that, if others have not experienced us expressing emotion before, they may feel confused or threatened, and it may take a while for them to adjust. Moreover, learning to express our emotions may take some working on – like any skill, it may feel difficult, awkward or unnatural. Again, if we persevere with our practice and our compassionate intention to help ourselves, expressing difficult emotions is likely to become easier and more natural for us.

Chapter summary

In this chapter we've explored difficulties in how we understand and experience our emotions, and ways in which our compassionate mind skills can help us work through these.

What we have learnt together	My personal reflections on the chapter
1. We can struggle with our emotions in a number of ways – these include difficulties in noticing, labelling, understanding and expressing emotions. 2. Learning to develop skills in these areas can help us better manage, or regulate, our emotions. 3. Our compassionate mind skills can help us to learn how to understand, validate, tolerate and express our feelings in a way that is helpful and adaptive.	

21 Putting our compassionate mind to work – Compassionate behaviour

'Nothing is predestined, the obstacles of your past can become the gateways that lead to new beginnings.'

– *Ralph Blum, The Book of Runes, 1932*

What is compassionate behaviour?

Just as with our attention, thinking and emotions, our behaviour (what we do, and the way we act towards ourselves and others) is also vulnerable to being captured by our threat system. When this happens, we can become engaged in behaviour that brings distress or difficulty into our lives, and at times into others people's lives too. For example, when stuck in anxiety, we may avoid doing things that we know would help us, such as seeing people, applying for a new job, engaging in activities and hobbies, or going on a date. If we get caught in anger, we might get stuck in blaming other people, being aggressive or deliberately unhelpful in a passively aggressive way.

Compassionate behaviour is often courageous

In our experience one of the great misconceptions about compassion is that it always involves being nice, kind and loving. Of course, compassion *can* involve these attributes, and these may guide our compassionate behaviours in a helpful and appropriate way. For example, the prototype of a compassionate person, someone who helps others who are struggling, would often bring to mind qualities of kindness and care. However, there is more to compassion than this. As the definition implies (as we explored in Chapter 5), compassion involves actively facing situations that cause distress for the purpose of alleviating suffering. To be able to do this we often need strength and courage, as engaging with distress can often be difficult and threatening in itself. Moreover, as we explored in Chapter 5, we can engage in compassionate acts without necessarily experiencing feelings of warmth and kindness towards others. For example, you may offer to help someone who has fallen even if you don't really like them or feel affection for them. Your action is guided by the intention to be supportive and alleviate pain, which can bypass feelings of warmth and liking.

This is an important concept to hold in mind. Whilst certain positive feelings can be present when engaging in compassionate behaviours, these are not necessary prerequisites of compassionate behaviour. Instead, qualities like strength and courage are often central in compassionate behaviours, particularly when compassion involves us engaging in things that are difficult, distressing or even threatening in some way.

It is important that our self-compassion is also underpinned by strength and compassion. Consider the following example: Steph has experienced social anxiety for most of her adult life, and it is now so severe that she often avoids seeing her friends or going to any social events. Recently, she has been invited to her best friend's thirtieth birthday party. Her friend has had a difficult year after losing her job and breaking up with her partner, and is really worried that no one will turn up to her party. Steph cares deeply about her friend and really wants to be there for her, but feels very anxious about the idea of being at a party, and considers making an excuse and not going. What would self-compassion involve in this situation for Steph?

> Having a nice bubble bath, glass of wine and watching a good film to make herself feel better for not going to her friend's birthday?
>
> or
>
> Trying to use the skills of her compassionate self (particularly commitment and strength) to tolerate her fears so that she can make it to the party, even for a short time?

It probably goes without saying then that self-compassion is not about being 'nice' to ourselves in a way that maintains our difficulties, stops us from taking responsibility or keeps us away from things that are important to us. Whilst it is understandable that Steph found the idea of going to the party very difficult, self-compassion here would involve her finding the courage to face up to (rather than avoid) her difficulties in order to overcome them, as well as being the type of friend she wanted to be. So, in the weeks running up to the party, Steph spent time engaging in things she found anxiety provoking (such as interacting with people more) in order to build up her confidence. She also practised skills in order to strengthen her compassionate mind (see Sections III, IV and V, pages 99–217). Of course, we are not saying that being kind to oneself – using relaxation (e.g. a warm bath) and nice things (e.g. nice food or watching a good film) cannot be examples of self-compassion. Rather, we want to emphasise the importance of confronting difficult situations (instead of burying ourselves underneath them) with self-compassion.

To further explore what compassionate behaviour is, and what it is not, take a look at the table below.

Compassionate behaviour is ...	Compassionate behaviour is not ...
Using our wisdom to guide: • Being supportive and encouraging towards ourselves, and other people who may be having difficulties • Facing our fears with kindness and strength • Engaging in the things that we find difficult in life, with courage • Learning to be assertive • Being able to share our feelings, concerns and needs • Tolerating feeling vulnerable.	• Saying 'yes' to other people, or being nice to them in order just to please them, or ensure they don't reject us • Hiding how we truly feel • Punishing ourselves • Giving in to others (this is submissive rather than assertive behaviour) • Doing 'nice' things for ourselves and others • Apologising for everything • Taking undue responsibility for things • Not feeling vulnerable.

Compassion has many faces

As we've seen in other sections of this book, compassion does not come in the form of 'one size fits all'. It can come with different combinations of qualities depending on the situation – for example, kindness, care, warmth, sensitivity, commitment, authority, wisdom, strength, courage and/or confidence. As we become more skilful in accessing our compassionate mind, we begin to understand what version of compassion we need at any moment, particularly the type of compassionate behaviour that would be helpful. These could range from listening and being available to actively comforting, encouraging and reassuring; to protecting, setting boundaries, and being firm; to relaxing and allowing ourself to rest from trying to achieve things; to facing something difficult or anxiety provoking. Below we will explore different types of compassionate behaviour, and how we might start to practise these.

Compassionate behaviour: Learning about what we avoid, and why we avoid it

Many psychological therapies see avoidance of difficulties as understandable, but also see avoidance as a contributing factor that often maintains problems. For example, if we are afraid of dogs, it is understandable that we may want to avoid being close to, or even seeing them. We sometimes refer to this avoidance as a 'safety' or 'protective' behaviour. It is linked to the threat system, and functions as a way of keeping us safe from something that we experience (or perceive) to be dangerous. However, our avoidance does not help us overcome our fears – in this case of dogs – as it does not reduce our underlying anxiety. Even if we became the best avoider of dogs in the world, this would not help us to deal with, or reduce the actual problem – fear of dogs. In fact, what we do know is that avoidance has the unintended consequence of fuelling our fears by confirming them. That is, the more we avoid dogs and feel the relief from doing so, the more we are likely to learn that it was in staying away from them that we felt better (i.e. a reduction in anxiety), which in turn can feed back in to our belief that they are dangerous and in need of staying away from. This can then continue in a vicious cycle. Let's spend some time exploring this idea in more detail, using Jacob's story as an example.

> *Example:* Jacob has been single for five years. In a previous relationship he was the victim of domestic violence and, subsequently, has found it difficult to become close to people. Although motivated to develop friendships and romantic relationships, he is anxious that he will be hurt and rejected if he allows himself to feel close to others. Over the years, he has turned down countless social invitations, opportunities to develop friendships and dates. Understandably, he now feels very lonely, low in confidence and depressed. He would like to be closer to people, but currently, feels overwhelmed by feelings of anxiety and shame, and he criticises himself for these difficulties.

It can be helpful if we take a few moments to think about the type of things we avoid in life. Think about this for yourself. These could be relationships, social situations, or interactions with other people, work tasks (e.g. giving presentations). They could be certain places or things, such as lifts, planes, heights, dogs, or the dark. Or they could be internal experiences – for example, certain difficult emotions or unpleasant memories. You may find it helpful to take a look back at the formulation you developed in Chapter 4, as the second and third columns might give you a clue about your fears (see pages 48–52). Let's look at this further by completing Worksheet 21.1.

Worksheet 21.1: What do I tend to avoid?

To start with, spend some time thinking about the things or situations you feel nervous about and tend to avoid (e.g. certain emotions, memories, people, places or situations).

_____

_____

_____

_____

Jacob's answer – 'I have avoided getting close to people. Work colleagues, potential friends or romantic partners. I fear I'll get hurt if I get close to people.'

How do you try and protect yourself from the things you fear? What are your safety or avoidance strategies?

_____

_____

_____

_____

Jacob's answer – 'I avoid eye contact and having conversations. I often say "no" to social opportunities, or make up excuses.'

What are you afraid might happen if you don't engage in your safety behaviours/avoidance?

_____

_____

_____

Jacob's answer – 'I think I will mess up and that people will not like me. I think other people will see I'm weak and take advantage of me.'

Now that you understand a bit more about the nature of your avoidance, it can be helpful to use your compassionate mind to connect with, and validate this. Use Worksheet 21.2 to help you with this.

Worksheet 21.2: Validating and tolerating fears and avoidance

Sit in a comfortable and upright position. Take a few moments to engage with your soothing rhythm breathing (see pages 124–28). Bring to mind the qualities of your compassionate self – care and commitment, strength and wisdom. Spend a little time feeling your way into this version of you. From this part of you, bring to mind the things that you find threatening, and the safety or avoidance strategies you use to manage these. As your compassionate self, take some time to reflect and make some notes on the following points:

Can you validate and have empathy for your fears, and crucially, the avoidant strategies you've been using to try and manage these? Is there a way of seeing that it makes sense that you may feel like this, given your fears? You may be able to make some notes on this, perhaps start by writing: It is understandable that I respond like this because …

_____

_____

_____

_____

Jacob's answer – 'It is understandable that I feel fearful like this because I have been withdrawing from people for so long now. I started to avoid people in the first place because I was hurt badly by someone in the past. My tricky brain goes in to threat mode telling me I am in danger.'

What might help me to tolerate, rather than avoid, my fear?

_____

_____

_____

_____

Jacob's answer – 'My compassionate self is strong and courageous and can help me tolerate my fear and face it. My compassionate self is committed and wants the best for me, and that involves developing relationships and getting closer to people. My compassionate self knows that learning new skills will take time and practice, and encourages me to continue to face my fears even if I find it difficult at times.'

Compassionate behaviour: bringing change to things we find difficult

Many of us recognise that in order to bring about change in our life, we need to change our behaviour. For example, we know that to get fit, we need to go to the gym or play more sport. We know that if we want to become good at playing the guitar, we need to practise regularly. If we want to change our job, we need to start looking at jobs that are available, get our CV up to date, and prepare for interviews. Whilst all of these are true, changing our behaviour to bring about positive change in our lives is by no means straightforward, or easy. Often, whilst we logically know what would be helpful to do, we continue to avoid making changes or procrastinate.

There may be many explanations for this; one common reason people struggle to change their behaviour, even when this is what they want, is because change is *difficult* and *effortful*, and our fears are often overwhelming or seemingly insurmountable obstacles. An aspect of psychological therapy often involves helping people engage with, and face their fears. This process is sometimes called 'exposure training'. The person is exposed to their feared situation (or object) in a gradual but repeated fashion and learns how to face and tolerate this in a way that lessens the power of the fear, and the need to avoid the situation. It has been found that, over time, this process tends to reduce levels of anxiety and fear. Compassionate Mind Training (CMT) takes a very similar position, and sees the development of a compassionate mind as a way to help us notice and understand our avoidance, whilst finding the strength, wisdom and commitment to face the things we fear, rather than avoid them. Let's take a look at how our compassionate minds can help us with these types of difficulties.

Exercise 1: Using Your Compassionate Mind to Work With Difficulties

Sit in a comfortable and upright position. Take a few moments to engage with your soothing rhythm breathing, helping your body to slow down a little. Bring to mind the qualities of your compassionate self – caring-commitment, strength and wisdom. Spend a little time feeling your way into this version of you.

From this part of you, take some time to think through each of the following questions, making notes below if that helps:

- What problems can you envisage experiencing if you begin to drop your protective (avoidance) strategies?

- What might get in the way of your desire to change?

- What can you do to support yourself with these difficulties?

- If you weren't afraid, what would be the first steps you'd be taking?

- If you had your compassionate self or compassionate other by your side, what would you be doing, and where could you start from?

- Remind yourself of why it is important to bring change to this area of your life – what important things would you be doing in life if you could manage your fears differently?

Notes and self-reflection:

_____

_____

_____

_____

Box 21: Tips on working with the common difficulties experienced with compassionate behaviour

Tips – working with the common difficulties experienced with compassionate behaviour

- Try to notice the threat system. Validate that it is trying to protect you, but use your compassionate mind skills (mindfulness, breathing, imagery) to help you anchor yourself back into the present, and to tolerate what has been activated

- If a friend was struggling with these difficulties, what would you advise them to do first?

- Remember to be caring and kind to yourself, and go at your own pace – small steps are often the most helpful when it comes to making changes

- The compassionate self understands and supports you, and most importantly, knows that change is hard but will encourage you as you work on this

- Try to compassionately respond to any threat thoughts and emotions that arise; validate them and return your attention to your intention to help yourself

- Turning your mind to a compassionate focus requires practice

- Make a commitment to behave in ways that help you move forward. This may mean acknowledging that in the short term things might be challenging

- Can you ask a friend, family member, colleague or partner to help you?

Compassionate behaviour – Facing our fears in a step-by-step way

Once we know what our avoidance and fears are about, and we can validate and understand them, we can begin taking the first steps towards change. Let's think about *how* we're going to do this. To start with, remind yourself about what you wrote earlier in the chapter (Worksheet 21.1) about the things you avoid in life, and would like to bring change to (see page 270).

Our next step would be to identify the things you might need to do, to help you face your fears. For example, TJ had a fear of public speaking. This was something he really wanted to work on because his boss had told him that he was ready for a promotion and that the new role involved leading meetings and giving regular presentations. TJ created a list of gradual steps, from the easiest task (preparing a presentation) to the most difficult (and dreaded) one (giving a presentation to the managers at work). He took his time to engage in and practise each step, and gradually worked his way up to his main goal. With each step he engaged his compassionate mind to deal with any fears or difficulties that got in the way of moving forward.

TJ's feared situations

1. Preparing for the presentation (e.g. research)

2. Writing the presentation

3. Practising the presentation in front of a mirror

4. Practising the presentation in front of my family

5. Practising the presentation in front of my friends

6. Presenting to friends at work

7. Presenting to managers at work

Like TJ, let's see if you can spend some time identifying some of the steps you might need to engage in, in order to face a difficulty or work towards a desired change. If you can, start at the bottom of Worksheet 21.3 (below) with those things that are easier, building up to the most difficult activity, or behaviour you would like to engage in to bring about the change that you want.

Worksheet 21.3: List of situations I want to face (from least anxiety-provoking to most challenging)

Activity
1.
2.
3.
4.
5.
6.
7.
8.

Now that we have an outline of some of the specific behaviours you are struggling with, it can be helpful to look at how we can engage in this using our compassionate mind.

Using imagery to help me prepare for change

Before you start to face your fears in 'real' life, it can be helpful to gradually work through your list of fears using your imagination. This is often referred to as *imaginal exposure*, starting with the situation that is the least anxiety provoking first. For example, if you are fearful of flying, it might be that you bring an image of your compassionate self to mind, going through different stages of what scares you most about this. So, you might imagine – the compassionate self with its wisdom, strength and commitment – managing and tolerating the process of checking-in at the baggage drop, going through security, getting on the plane and so on.

Exercise 2: Using Imagery to Help Me Gradually Face My Fears

Sit in an upright position, and engage in your soothing rhythm breathing and friendly facial expression (see pages 122–28). Allow your breathing to slow a little, and gently rest your attention in the flow of breathing in and breathing out. When you feel ready, bridge in to your compassionate self and its qualities of caring-commitment, wisdom and strength. Allow yourself to embody these qualities – notice your facial expressions, body posture and compassionate intent.

As your compassionate self, now imagine engaging in the least anxiety-provoking situation on your list (Worksheet 21.3). Imagine yourself in the situation, engaging in the behaviour that you find difficult or anxiety provoking, from the part of you that is strong, wise and has a commitment to engage in things that are beneficial for you. Notice if your threat system kicks in as you're engaging in this imagery. If this happens, remember that your compassionate self is strong, confident and wise, and can work with this too. Tap back in to the bodily sense of your compassionate self – your body posture, facial expression and vocal tone. Use your soothing breathing and body posture to ground yourself before returning to the scenario in your mind's eye. Once you have finished taking this imaginary journey as your compassionate self, return to your soothing breathing. It may help to spend some time in your safe place before you let the image fade.

Self-reflection: What was this exercise like? How strong was your threat response throughout? How did your compassionate self help you work through this?

_____

_____

_____

_____

Over the coming days and weeks, take your time to work slowly through your list, moving towards the most difficult activity when you feel ready. Continue to use your compassionate mind skills to help you with this, and with any difficulties or struggles you have.

Taking action – real-life exposure

Whilst using imagery is a powerful and often helpful way of beginning to approach things we're avoiding, this is, of course, not a substitute for actually engaging in these things in real life. This merely provides a template for how we can go about doing this, and the steps involved.

Look back at your list and consider whether you need to break it down further into smaller steps. What would be the first step you could take to begin to face this challenge in real life? Everybody's list will be different. If you have a fear of heights, for example, your first exposure exercise might be to look out of a window on the second floor of a building. If you have a phobia of dogs, the first step might be to watch the film *Lassie*!

Self-reflection: What would help you to prepare to take action? How could your compassionate self help you here? What qualities of your compassionate self would be important to support you? What words of encouragement would motivate and empower you to begin to take some steps towards overcoming your fears?

_____

_____

_____

_____

Exercise 3: Engaging in Compassionate Action

Putting your compassion into action involves starting with the least challenging step. See if you can practise this first step for a while until you feel better able to tolerate your anxiety and this begins to dissipate a little. Move on to the next step when you feel ready. With each step that you take remember to first spend time bringing your compassionate mind 'online' to encourage you to face and continue to work on each step. Take time to work through your listed steps in a gradual way and persevere with the support of your compassionate mind. Try to give yourself credit for what you are able to do, even if you feel this didn't go perfectly. Remember, we all have setbacks – they are part of the human experience.

Self-reflection: How did you find engaging in your difficulties in this gradual, step-by-step manner?

_____

_____

_____

Working with setbacks

It's common for people to experience setbacks and difficulties when they start to approach the things they previously avoided because of the difficulties involved. Frequently, we make attempts to engage in a difficult behaviour or action, but then we can feel overwhelmed or disheartened, and step back from our efforts. Other times we engage in the new behaviour but become critical of ourselves – 'I didn't do that well enough' or 'I'm so weak for struggling with this; I shouldn't be finding it so hard and should not be in this situation in the first place'. It is in these moments when we are struggling not only with the behaviour itself, but with our critical minds too, that we particularly need compassion. We can use such setbacks, or 'slips' in our progress as opportunities to engage our compassionate minds, to support ourselves to carry on and move towards valued goals. Here are some ideas of what to do:

Spend a few moments engaging in your soothing rhythm breathing (see pages 124–28) and then connect with your ideal compassionate self/other. From this perspective, turn towards the setback/disappointment and consider the following:

- Try and be aware and notice the feeling you're having (e.g. disappointment, shame, anger)

- Try and validate why you're feeling like this. Consider using a Compassionate Thought Record (see Chapter 19, page 245) and spend some time considering alternative or more balanced perspectives to the situation, bringing a sense of understanding and empathy towards yourself. For example, reminding yourself that 'this is not my fault', that these are understandably difficult things to do and that many others struggle to engage with anxiety-provoking situations and behaviours too.

- Consider what would help you going forward. What can you learn from this? What would help you next time? Do you need to practise anything that may increase your chances of overcoming this next step?

Self-reflection: What was it like trying to bring your compassionate mind to the setback/ struggle? What impact did this have on your feelings, and your motivation to re-engage in the difficult behaviour?

Compassionate Planning: Pre, During and After (The Compassion PDA)

One way to bring together what we've discussed so far is to develop a Compassion PDA. PDA stands for the 'pre', 'during' and 'after' stages of engaging in something that we find threatening. One way of approaching the tougher things in life is to think like a sportswoman or man. Let's imagine that Usain Bolt or Serena Williams is focused on doing well in a big event. One way they could focus on this would be to consider what would be helpful for them before the event happens (pre), as the event is happening (during), and once the event has finished (after).

For example, it might be that before the event they prepare by doing lots of fitness training (running, lifting weights in the gym), and eating healthily. They might also work hard on training on specific aspects of their sport (e.g. how to start well in racing, or serve in tennis), as well as making tactical plans for how they are going to manage the event when it comes around. On the day of the event, they might engage in specific behaviours and activities to prepare their bodies (e.g. eating certain foods, resting, warming up and stretching) and minds (for example, imagining how they are going to compete, or using encouraging inner 'self-talk'). After the event, there's also work to be done; they would need to warm down to minimise the risk of injury, and then review their performance with their coach, and consider what they can learn and take forward in a wise way for the future.

It turns out that we can take a similar approach to working with things in our own life. Let's explore this with the example of Annette, who came to therapy struggling with anxiety and in particular, with going for interviews and giving presentations. With her therapist, she explored the concept of the Compassion PDA, and together they developed the following:

Annette's Compassion PDA

Difficulty	Pre	During	After
Going for a job interview. I panic about it for weeks ahead, and clam up during the interview. Afterwards, I feel very angry and critical with myself, and I play over and over what I've done wrong.	It's helpful to spend more time practising mindfulness and soothing rhythm breathing – this will help me to calm my mind and research what I need to know, and prepare my answers. I'll also have a trial interview with my colleague and friend Mason.	On the day I'll do some breathing practice to start with. Before I go into the interview, I'm going to try to embody my compassionate self – posture and voice tone. When I'm in the interview, I'm going to use my soothing rhythm breathing to slow down.	It's probably best that I speak to a friend, rather than sit on my own. I will remind myself that I am doing well facing my anxiety and fears. It might be helpful to write down my answers, so that I can go over them on another day. It might also be useful to write a compassionate letter to myself about the interview and how I did.

See if you can take the same approach with something that you're finding difficult. To do this, you can use Worksheet 21.4. To start with, write down in the first column the situation that you're finding difficult. Then, as we've done throughout many of the recent chapters, spend some time getting in contact with the part of you that can helpfully direct your PDA – your compassionate self. From this wise, strong and caring part, take your time to think through what might help before, during and after facing this challenge.

1. Pre: Try to consider what steps you could take that would help in the lead-up to engaging in this difficulty. Are there things that could help you prepare for this event (e.g. things you need to find out, or learn, or things you could practise?). Are there things you could look out for so that you could do them less (e.g. catastrophising or criticising yourself)? Are there any skills that you've practised in this workbook that might support you?

2. During: Try to consider what would help you to actually 'do' the thing you find difficult at the time. Would it be helpful to have some support from a friend? Could you use your compassionate self to do this? Can your breathing help you at all?

3. After: What would be helpful for you after you faced the situation? If it's gone well, what would be a wise thing to do? How can your compassionate self help you to hold on to, savour and learn from the 'positives'? If it hasn't gone so well, what would help you to tolerate the disappointment, sadness or anxiety that might emerge? What could you learn from this for the future? What would prevent you from getting caught up in self-criticism or unhelpful rumination?

Remember to praise yourself for facing your anxieties. For many people we've worked with, the PDA has become an essential supportive tool to engage in actions that are challenging. If you can, try it out initially with two or three different scenarios. As you get more confident using the idea, it's likely you'll be able to develop more in-depth, and nuanced PDAs.

Worksheet 21.4: The Compassion PDA

Difficulty	Pre	During	After

Self-reflection: How did you find developing and using your Compassion PDA? How did it help you to plan and carry out a difficult task? Is there anything you would do differently next time you faced your fears?

_____

_____

_____

Compassionate behaviour: Seeking support and care

So far in this chapter we have been discussing compassionate behaviours that involve us managing our difficulties on our own. Whilst these are helpful steps, we would not want our efforts to be at the expense of being open to the support and help of others. In our experience, many of us can be blocked in seeking help when we experience distress and suffering, and this is particularly the case when we experience shame and self-criticism (we will explore these concepts further in Chapter 23). Often it is exactly the support and encouragement of others (who are, of course, compassionate!) that can help us to feel safe enough to engage in things that are scary and difficult. So just as we explored in Chapter 16 (pages 207–12), being open to the care, support and compassion of others can in itself be a type of self-compassionate behaviour and can also help us to manage things that we may have otherwise avoided, or felt overwhelmed by.

Example: Eli felt a lump on her breast whilst showering. Immediately, she felt terrified that she might have cancer, and began to read articles on the internet about her likely prognosis, and a number of unpleasant treatment options. She quickly felt overwhelmed, anxious and like her life had already ended. Following this, she experienced an urge to ignore these worries, to push them out of her mind, and just 'get on with things'. In fact, for three days she carried on with life, going to work and did not tell anyone. Whenever she thought about the lump she tried to distract herself and push the worries from her mind. However, she knew, deep down, that this was avoiding the reality of the situation. Although she found it hard, using her compassionate self she found the strength and courage to meet with her best friend Lola. Lola was supportive – she listened to Eli calmly, validated her fears and after many hugs and encouraging words, the two of them booked Eli an appointment to see a doctor to get the lump checked out.

The key thing about this example is that although hard, Eli was able to turn to the care, support and compassion of her friend, who helped her then to tolerate her own threat system (anxiety and avoidance), and encouraged her to take steps to do something about her suffering. Let's have a think about how this could work for you.

> *Exercise 3: Seeking Help From Others*
>
> Spend a few moments reconnecting with your soothing rhythm breathing, and when you feel ready, bridge in to your compassionate self, and its qualities of caring-commitment, wisdom and strength. Allow yourself to embody these qualities – to notice your facial expressions, body posture and compassionate intent. When you feel ready, from this compassionate part of you, consider the following questions, making notes as you go along.

Self-reflection: Who might help me to manage my difficulties? Who could I turn to, or seek help from, given the difficulties I'm going through?

_____

_____

What are my threat thoughts and feelings about approaching / asking this person for support?

_____

_____

What would help me to manage my threat system so that I can approach someone for help and support? How could my compassionate mind skills help me here?

_____

_____

_____

What steps can I take now to seek out help?

_____

_____

_____

If you did manage to seek support from others about one of your struggles, what was this like? What did you gain from this? What would help you to do this again in the future?

_____

_____

_____

_____

What have you learnt from the above exercise?

_____

_____

Being assertive

Many of us have had that moment when we've really wanted to stand up to someone, ask for something or express an opinion, but rather than doing so, we've kept our mouth shut and remained silent. Equally, some of us often find it difficult to say 'no' and can find ourselves engaging in things we don't really want to do, or going along with someone else's wishes. Being assertive involves finding respectful ways to voice our thoughts, feelings and needs and expressing ourselves in a way that may be beneficial to us, and, ideally, to the person we're communicating with.

Many people find assertiveness tricky. Some people, rather than expressing their views, needs and wishes assertively, respond in a passive or submissive way. Others struggle with the other extreme of expression, and communicate aggressively, making angry demands, blaming, and even threatening other people.

Example: Tara had been in a relationship with Mark for three years. She loved him very much, and in many ways felt very happy in their relationship. However, as someone who was introverted and at times shy and quiet, she found it difficult to express her needs and what she wanted with Mark, who was naturally a very confident, outgoing and dominant personality. Recently, she had started to feel taken for granted, ignored and even resentful after Mark made a number of decisions on their behalf without consulting with her. After talking to a friend about how she was feeling, Tara realised that, although it was understandable to be annoyed with Mark, she also needed to take responsibility for her part in this and learn to respond to her wishes and opinions. She was able to see how she was used to saying 'Yes, sure, I don't mind' to many things (including where to go for dinner) when she actually had a specific view or preference.

When we start to think about how to be assertive, there are a number of steps that can help. We'll use Tara as an example in each of these.

1. Identifying situations where you struggle being assertive

Take a little time to think about your life, and the things you find difficult to be assertive about. Maybe this is linked to sharing your feelings with someone, or expressing your preferences, or asking for what you want. Perhaps you find it difficult to ask other people to do things for you, or to stick up for your view (e.g. with a boss, colleague or friend). Make a few notes below about what you find difficult.

_____

_____

_____

2. Looking for what sits behind non-assertiveness

It can be useful to consider some of the reasons behind our difficulties with assertiveness. Take a few minutes to think over what stops you from being assertive. Is there a fear about what might happen if you start behaving in a more assertive way? Maybe a fear about the person you would become? Do you have any concern about how others may respond to you (i.e. in a negative way) if you start being more assertive? Make a few notes below:

_____

_____

_____

Tara's answer – 'I'm scared that if I starting saying what I want, other people will think I'm selfish and demanding. I think that Mark might not like it and would not want to be around me.'

3. Bringing compassion to our difficulty – being assertive

Take a moment to get back in the shoes of your compassionate self (or connect with your compassionate other), and its commitment, strength and wisdom. From this part of you, how might you bring compassion to this struggle to be assertive? Are there emotions, such as anxiety, shame or guilt, making this tough? How could your compassionate self validate, have empathy for, or be supportive towards this difficulty you're having?

_____

_____

_____

Tara's answer – 'My compassionate self knows this is very difficult for me, and helps me to understand that it's not my fault. I can see that this is a similar way that my mum is with my dad and her friends. My compassionate self wants to support me with this difficulty.'

4. Finding the language of assertiveness

Before we actually engage in more assertive communication, it can be helpful to plan what we might say. There are different ways to do this, but as ever, it's helpful to do this from your compassionate self. So take a minute or two to connect with your strength, commitment and wisdom. Consider what you could say to the other person, as your compassionate self.

From this part of you, see if you can answer the following:

What do you need? (What needs or feelings would you like to express?). Try starting this with 'I would like …', 'I need …', 'I feel …' or 'I think …'.

_____

_____

Tara's answer – 'I need to be able to voice my own feelings and needs, to share the things I would like to do.'

Why is this important for you? ('This is important for me because …')

_____

_____

Tara's answer – 'This is important for me because I want to feel closer to you, but for this to be based on an equal, shared and balanced relationship in which we both contribute equally.'

What would you like the person to do? (For example, how would you like them to behave towards you?) This might start with 'I would like you to …'

_____

_____

Tara's answer – 'I would like you to think about me more often. Even if I'm quiet, it's still important to remember that I have thoughts and ideas about things.'

So as to not push the other person away, or come across as too aggressive, or demanding, it can be helpful once you've voiced your 'assertiveness' to ask the other person whether they are willing to talk about this further; how you would really appreciate it – and them – if this was the case.

5. Being assertive – using the compassionate self

It might be important to find a way to put assertiveness into action now – to translate the words you outlined above and find a helpful way to communicate these to the other person. Perhaps spend some time focusing your intention on when you're going to do this and who you're going to do this with. As we've looked at before, think about how your compassionate self might help you to plan for this, and make a few notes below on this.

_____

_____

_____

6. Managing setbacks

Although learning to be assertive can be tricky, over time you may notice that you feel more able or confident to do this. As we've reflected upon in previous chapters, it might be that you experience setbacks or difficulties whilst practising assertiveness, and we'd encourage you here to turn back to your compassionate self as a way of helping you to manage this. You may also find it helpful to use a Compassionate Thought Form (Chapter 19, page 245), or take a look through the next chapter on compassionate letter writing as a way to support yourself.

Chapter summary

In this chapter we've explored how our compassionate mind might help us to behave or act in ways that are helpful for us.

What we have learnt together	My personal reflections on the chapter
1. The way we behave can be influenced by our threat system.	
2. Compassionate behaviour is not just about being 'nice' or 'kind' – it involves cultivating and using qualities (wisdom, strength and commitment) to act in ways that will be helpful to us, and others.	
3. Compassionate behaviour often involves strength and courage to do things that we find difficult.	
4. It can be helpful for us to learn how to break down difficult actions into smaller steps, to seek support (from our compassionate self and compassionate people in our life), and to be caring, kind and encouraging towards ourselves.	
5. We can use our compassionate mind skills to learn how to assert ourselves, and express our needs to others.	

22 Compassionate mind – Bringing together the whole – Compassionate letter writing

'Our greatest glory consists not in never falling, but in rising every time we fall.'

– Oliver Goldsmith

In this chapter we will look at another way that you can put your 'compassion into action'. We will explore how using writing may be a helpful way of engaging a variety of compassionate skills – attention, thinking, and behaviour – to support you in managing difficulties.

Letter writing

For millennia, people from diverse cultures have found that writing – whether in the form of a journal, diary, poetry or letters – is a useful way of reflecting on difficulties, and finding ways to manage struggles. Writing about our problems seems to help put them in perspective. As one client told us, writing things down 'takes the pain out of my head, and out onto the paper – this helps me to get it organised and see it more clearly'. Research seems to back this up. The American psychologist, James W. Pennebaker, found that writing about things that we struggle with, such as stresses, strains or difficult events in life, could have a positive effect upon our physical and psychological health over time.

Compassionate letter writing

In Compassionate Mind Training (CMT) we use Pennebaker's insights but, as you can probably guess, add a slight twist! That is, we learn how to write about our difficulties from our compassionate minds, the part of us that can bring a sensitivity to suffering (first psychology of compassion), and have the wisdom and motivation to find ways to cope with and alleviate these (second psychology of compassion). So, compassionate letter writing is a way of bringing together many of the compassionate skills – attention, thinking, emotion and behaviour, which we have been working on in the workbook.

There are different ways we can write compassionate letters. The general purpose of compassionate letter writing is to:

- Express concern, non-judgement and genuine caring to ourselves

- Demonstrate sensitivity to our pain and suffering

- Help us to be more tolerant of our distress and difficulties

- Help us to understand and have empathy for our struggles.

Box 22.1 offers some hints and prompts for you to consider before we get started.

Tips – compassionate letter writing

- Try to find a quiet, safe place where you will not be disturbed

- Experiment using the first person (I) and the second person (you). Many people find it harder using the first person, e.g. 'I can see that this is not my fault, I have done the best I can' rather than the second person, e.g. 'This is not your fault, you have done the best you can'. Explore which you find easier, and use that to start with

- Your letters do not need to be perfect. The purpose of this exercise is really in the intention to approach something that you're struggling with, supported by the qualities of compassion – for example, care, empathy and support

- It is OK to go back and change your letter – but try not to get too caught up in fine detail, or trying to make it 'perfect'

- As you write, keep a mindful eye on which 'part' of you is writing the letter – sometimes we can start the letter with a very compassionate voice, but quickly move to a cold, critical or demanding voice

- One size does not fit all. See if you can play around with your compassionate letter writing. We have provided a structure to start you off, but feel free to find your own style, over time

- It may be helpful to re-read your letters on a weekly, or monthly basis. Some of the people we work with like to audio record their letters and listen to them. If you do record your letter, try to read it out loud with a warm, caring voice tone.

Exercise 1: Compassionate Letter Writing

We're going to spend some time in this next section guiding you to writing a compassionate letter. In all, there are ten steps to this approach. Although it can be helpful to take them in order, this isn't fixed. This order is simply a guide for how you can structure the letter writing process. Don't worry too much at this stage if you get stuck at one step, it's OK to move on to the next one. We will use Joe as an example throughout.

Example: Joe came to therapy looking for help with feeling anxious and low in mood. He had been made redundant from his job a couple of months earlier, and was feeling deeply ashamed and low in self-worth because of this. To try to manage some of his feelings, he had been drinking far more than normal. He noticed that he was having more arguments with friends and family members.

Step 1: Engage your compassionate mind

As you might be able to guess, the first step in letter writing involves helping you to connect with a part of you that is going to write the letter – your compassionate self. Now, you can also choose to write your letter from the perspective of your ideal compassionate other, but for the purpose of this letter, we are going to draw upon your compassionate self. To do this, first find a quiet place to sit and, with an upright body posture, spend a few moments mindfully connecting with your soothing rhythm breathing (see pages 124–28). When you feel ready, spend a little time connecting with the qualities of your ideal compassionate self – your caring-commitment, wisdom and strength. You may find it helpful to read back through the guidelines for this practice in Chapter 12 (pages 167–83). When you feel connected with your compassionate self, move on to Step 2.

Step 2: Motivation – Why am I writing this letter?

Before writing anything, it is helpful to tune in to your motivation for writing. Having connected with your compassionate self, see if you can focus on your intention to convey your compassion through this letter, in order to be helpful, supportive and encouraging with regards to a difficulty you may be facing. Spend thirty seconds, or so just holding this in the front of your mind, before you move on to Step 3.

Step 3: Beginning the letter and identifying a difficulty

So, to start the letter, we need to do two things:

- Direct the letter to yourself

- Identify a problem, or difficulty, that you are struggling (or have struggled) with, that you will focus the letter on.

As this is a letter to yourself, see if you can start by greeting yourself. 'Dear (your name)' or 'Hello (your name)' are two options of how to use your name directly. Sometimes people prefer something slightly different, like: 'Dear me'. See what feels OK for you.

Following this, we need to start the letter with identifying what the struggle is. Joe's letter started as follows:

Dear Joe,

I know that life is difficult at the moment, as you have been struggling with the impact of being made redundant, and you have been feeling very critical with yourself and hopeless about your future.

Step 4: Validation and empathy for the struggle

As we have explored in previous chapters, it can be helpful to validate and understand our feelings and struggles in life. So after outlining what the current struggle or difficulty is, it can be useful to turn our compassionate minds to understanding why we are feeling the way we are (in contrast to how many of us often respond to our distress through invalidation and confusion). Whilst connected with his compassionate self, Joe wrote the following:

It's understandable that you're feeling like you are. It's hard for anyone to lose their job, but especially after working there for so many years. You worked really hard in this role, and committed so much of your life to the company. It's also understandable that you feel like this, given your experiences in life – being raised to believe that you are only a good and worthy person if you work extremely hard. It also makes sense that you feel anxious about the future and whether the mortgage will get paid. You love your family more than anything in the world, and the last thing you ever wanted was to cause them any difficulties.

Step 5: Understanding of your attempts to manage your threat system – not your fault

As we explored in Chapter 4 on formulation (see pages 51–59), when our threat systems are triggered, we often engage in a variety of safety or protective behaviours to manage the threat. It can be helpful in your letters to outline the attempts you've made to manage your difficulties, and any negative consequences that arose from these attempts. Crucially it's important to see these consequences as unintended and 'not your fault'. This is what Joe wrote:

I know that you've been trying to manage your painful feelings of shame and anxiety by avoiding thinking about the situation and drinking more frequently. Unfortunately, this has brought some unintended problems, in particular arguments at home. It's not your fault that you've been trying to manage things this way, you were never taught any other ways of dealing with your feelings and you were just trying to find some way of helping yourself.

Step 6: Taking responsibility

Whilst it's not our fault that we get caught up in various safety strategies, it is our responsibility to develop the skills to manage these difficulties in a more helpful way. Here, it's often important to tap into the qualities of strength and wisdom, and our desire to approach things in a different, and more helpful way. Holding this in mind, Joe wrote:

Whilst it's not your fault for avoiding talking about what happened or for drinking more, it is important that you start to take responsibility for this, as the drinking is causing you more pain. It may be helpful if you engage your wisdom and strength, and begin to think about what you would like to do differently, and focus on your commitment to bring a different way of dealing with this difficult situation.

Step 7: Exploring how to help – compassionate thoughts and action

Now that you've started to commit to change and take responsibility, it can be helpful to see how your compassionate mind can help guide you through this difficulty and take steps towards change. If you look at Chapters 19 (pages 231–49) and 21 (pages 266–91) you will see more information on this. The intention here is to try and bring balance to your thinking, and engage in behaviours that are likely to help you face the difficulty, and bring some positive changes. Here, Joe wrote:

> Although you're blaming yourself for losing your job, it might be helpful to remember that you had a good review recently, so you can see that this is not a reflection on your skills. You can also see that it wasn't personal – a number of people lost their jobs and have also been struggling during the past couple of months as well. It might help to speak to them about how you are feeling. It might also be helpful to speak to Cassie about how to improve your CV, and start looking after your health again by cutting down on alcohol and doing some exercise.

Step 8: Working with blocks, difficulties and setbacks

It would be wonderful if our attempts to bring about change were smooth and successful, this is not always the case. It can be helpful in your letter to consider what difficulties or setbacks you might experience in your attempts to bring change. In thinking about this, Joe wrote:

> It might be helpful to keep an eye out for any times when you think you might need a drink, and plan for other things to do instead (for example, practise mindfulness, do some exercise, or meet with friends who don't drink). The main thing for you to keep in mind is the risk for you to want to bury your head in the sand if you start feeling more anxious and ashamed again. Try and keep a 'mindful eye' on this,

noticing your thoughts and feelings. This will give you an early warning about your tendency to revert back to familiar, but unhelpful, coping mechanisms, and guide you as to what to do differently to prevent this.

Step 9: Compassionate commitment to bringing change

In terms of writing, the final step is to convey a sense of your commitment to the process of change, or the process of supporting yourself in this. Joe wrote:

Please remember that I'll be there for you to help with all of this. Try to hold in mind your intention and commitment – to take steps to deal with this difficult situation in a different way, to focus on being the version of you that you want to be, the version that you will be proud of. Let's start with small steps. How about tomorrow you speak to Cassie about things and then we can take it from there? Remember, you're not on your own with this.

Step 10: Compassionate reading

When you have finished writing your letter, there is one final step: to read the letter back to yourself. You can do this out loud or in your head. Either way, the key is to read it from a particular part of you (your compassionate self, or compassionate other), and to do this with a warm, caring voice tone. It can also be important to take your time with this, reading the letter at a measured pace, rather than rushing through it. This will allow your mind to really hear and feel the words, feelings and intention behind the letter.

Having had a chance to read through the ten steps, don't feel you have to include every single one if they don't feel relevant. Perhaps just begin by finding a piece of paper and setting aside some time to have a go at writing about something you've been struggling with recently.

Box 22.2: Common difficulties and helpful hints with compassionate letter writing

Common difficulties	Helpful hints
It seems stupid to be writing letters to myself.	We know that some of these exercises can seem a little unnatural. If you can, do your best to try them a few times. It may be that over time you'll start to feel more at ease with this process, and it will become more comfortable.
The outline of the letter is difficult – there is a lot to remember.	Please remember that the outline we have given is only a guide. If this feels too complicated, just start with what you can. Ultimately, the most important part is to practise writing (and relating) to yourself from the compassionate part of you.
I don't know how to start the letter – it feels scary to even put pen to paper.	As with many things, the first step is the most difficult! It can be helpful to spend some extra time tuning in to your soothing rhythm breathing (see pages 124–28) and helping yourself to feel grounded. Try to focus on connecting with your compassionate self, and in particular the quality of strength and courage. Remember, there is not an absolutely 'right' letter, so try to experiment and play around with this process, if you can.
I started writing the letter in a compassionate way, but then I found that I began to be critical of myself.	This is common in the letter writing process – you're not the only one. Sometimes people describe the compassionate self as being like a battery – they charge it up, and it works for a while, but then it goes flat, and their self-critical part takes over. Taking a moment to reconnect and recharge your compassionate self is important. When you feel connected with your compassionate qualities again, see if you can return to writing the letter.

Chapter summary

In this chapter we've explored how compassionate letter writing can bring together a number of the skills we've been learning over the past few chapters, and apply them in a structured, written form.

What we have learnt together	My personal reflections on the chapter
1. Writing about how we feel can help us to work through difficulties we are experiencing. 2. Compassionate letters can involve a number of stages, including paying attention to a current difficulty, validating or having empathy for this, and finding ways of managing this in a new, more helpful way.	

SECTION VII

PUTTING OUR COMPASSIONATE MIND TO WORK WITH COMMON DIFFICULTIES

Although we've been working with how compassion may be a helpful guide to our attention, thinking, emotions and behaviour, there are some common difficulties that we can experience that go across these areas that often make life difficult. In this penultimate section of the workbook, we are going to explore how we can take the skills of our compassionate mind, and apply them to three areas of our lives:

- To our multiple – and often confusing – responses we can have to the same situation

- To experiences of shame and self-criticism

- To our fears and blocks to compassion.

23 Working with common difficulties – Understanding and bringing compassion to our multiple selves

'We meet ourselves time and again in a thousand disguises on the path of life.'

– Carl Jung

In Chapters 2 and 3 we introduced the idea of us having multiple selves or parts, but what do we mean when we talk about different parts of us? When we initially think about who we are – that is, the way we think, feel and act in the world – there can be a strong sense of a coherent, consistent 'whole' – a 'self' that stays the same throughout the day, week or year, regardless of what is happening around us. However, when we look at our experiences more closely we can begin to recognise that we have multiple and ever-changing emotional experiences, thoughts and urges, and engage in different behaviours and roles depending on what's happening around us, how we feel, where we are and what is expected of us. For example, if we narrowly escape being run over by a car that has skipped a red light, our anxious 'self' might show up, guiding our attention to danger, influencing our thinking ('The roads around here are so dangerous, I could have been killed') and our behaviour (being more cautious). However, it could also be that our angry part (or 'self') shows up and responds in a different way – focusing our attention and thoughts on the driver who almost killed us ('That stupid idiot, he could have killed me'), and guiding our actions to confront and challenge the transgressor (e.g. by shouting, waving a fist, or even chasing after the car to have a 'go' at the driver). These different emotional 'selves' sit within us, and each can influence our mind, how we feel in our body, and can impact on our actions in quite different ways.

One of the challenges that many of us face is being able to experience the different parts of us in a balanced and helpful way. Unfortunately, many of us can become stuck in just one self (e.g. angry or anxious) and this may limit flexible and healthy responses to what has happened/is happening. Moreover, as the different selves often have conflicting urges and needs in response to a situation, if we do experience more than one in close proximity to another, this can be rather unsettling. Think about the mixed feelings we can have when we are criticised in front of other people. A part of us might feel very angry at the person who has done this and want to lash out (verbally or physically); another part might feel nervous and want to run away or avoid being 'seen'; whilst another part might feel sad and hurt, and want to cry. All of these experiences and responses can ripple through us very quickly, and potentially leave us feeling confused, out of control or overwhelmed.

In this chapter, we are going to help you explore three different 'selves', linked to three of our primary emotions: anger, anxiety and sadness. We will do this through an exercise called 'multiple selves', in which we will explore these ideas in an experiential way, helping you to learn more about the different parts of you. For this exercise, we are going to use the example of an argument. After trying this, you might want to use a different example, such as something you feel you've failed at, a setback in life, or a situation in a relationship that you're struggling with. We will guide you through the exercise and illustrate with an example using Jasper's experience. Here is a bit of background about Jasper:

> *Example*: Jasper's story: Jasper is a 32-year-old man who came to therapy for help with controlling his anger. Recently, he had a big argument with one of his employees, Janet, after she made a mistake that cost the firm quite a lot of money. As a child, he described how his father and teachers had compared him negatively with his siblings, all of whom were A* students. Jasper recalled always feeling that he wasn't good enough.

Exercise: multiple selves

To start this exercise, bring to mind an argument or disagreement you had with someone, preferably recently, but if not, some time in the past. Spend a minute or so remembering what the argument was about, where you were, and who you were arguing with. See if you can choose an example that is currently not too activating for your mind, so your threat response doesn't get in the way of doing the exercise. If it helps, write a few notes about the argument below. When you have brought this experience to mind, see if you can move on to the next steps.

_____

_____

Step 1: Angry Part

See if you can bring to mind the part of you that felt angry about this argument. Allow yourself to feel into this part of yourself, letting go, if you can, of any other emotions or feelings you might have about what happened. When you feel connected to your angry part, go through the following steps, making a quick note at each step.

Thoughts: What thoughts does your angry part have about the argument? (What words or phrases come to mind? If it could speak, what would your angry part say?)

_____

_____

Jasper's answer – 'It took me ages to get that customer on board and now Janet has made a stupid mistake and messed it all up. She's an idiot.'

Body: Try to notice where in your body you can feel your angry part.

_____

Jasper's answer – 'I notice tightness in my chest, head and fists.'

Behaviour: If this angry part was in complete control, what would it want to do, given the situation? (For example, shout, complain, hit or smash something.)

_____

_____

Jasper's answer – 'I want to shout at her and smash her desk!'

Memories: Holding in mind your angry part, what memories come to mind?

_____

_____

Jasper's answer – 'I remember getting angry with my teacher when he told me that I wasn't as good as my sister.'

Outcome: What would help your angry part to settle? What does it need? What would it see as a good outcome to the argument?

_____

_____

Jasper's answer – 'She (Janet) needs to apologise to me for screwing things up and tell me that I'm right, and then work lots of hours overtime to make up for it.'

Once you've got 'into the skin' of your angry part, and completed the above, see if you can gently let it go, slowly allowing this part of you to ease away. Take a few slower breaths, feeling your way back in to a grounded, calm position.

Step 2: Anxious Part

This time, we're going to spend some time connecting with a part of you that was anxious about this argument. Allow yourself to feel into this part of yourself, taking your time. When you feel connected to your anxious part, take some time to think about the following questions, making a few notes at each step.

Thoughts: What thoughts does your anxious part have about the argument? (What words or phrases come to mind? If it could speak, what would your anxious part say?)

_____

_____

Jasper's answer – 'The company isn't going to survive, there's no way we can keep going at this rate.'

Body: Try to notice where in your body you can feel your anxious part (what physical sensations you experience).

Jasper's answer – 'Tension in my stomach, increased heart rate and shaky hands.'

Behaviour: If your anxious part was in complete control, what would it want to do, given the situation? (For example, run away, avoid the person, disappear or hide.)

Jasper's answer – 'My anxious part wants to run away and not have to deal with this.'

Memories: Holding in mind your anxious part, what memories come to mind?

Jasper's answer – 'I remember waiting to find out my exam results on my own, as my parents had gone away on holiday. I didn't do as well as I'd hoped, and dreaded them calling to find out how I'd done.'

Outcome: What would help your anxious part settle? What would it need? What would it see as a good outcome to the argument?

Jasper's answer – 'For this situation to be over and done with – for things to be back to the way they were before and for everything to be secure.'

Once you completed the above, see if you can gently come out of the 'skin' of your anxious part, and let that ease away. Take a few slower breaths, allowing your body to slow down. When you feel ready, move on to Step 3.

Step 3: Sad Part

Take a moment to bring to mind the part of you that felt sad about this argument. Allow yourself to step into the shoes of this part of yourself. When you feel connected to your sad part, go through the following questions, making a quick note after each one.

Thoughts: What thoughts does your sad part have about the argument? (What words or phrases come to mind? If it could speak, what would your sad part say?)

_____

_____

Jasper's answer – 'Janet was such a good friend. Now she'll keep her distance and I'll be on my own at work.'

Body: Try to notice where in your body can you feel your sad part.

_____

Jasper's answer – 'I feel a heaviness in my stomach and around my heart.'

Behaviour: If your sad part was in control, what would it want to do, given the situation? (For example, to give up, cry or seek reassurance?)

_____

_____

Jasper's answer – 'My sad part wants to curl up in a ball and cry.'

Memories: Holding in mind your sad part, what memories come to mind?

_____

_____

Jasper's answer – '*I just have a picture of me as a young boy, sat on my bed, feeling upset and crying after disappointing my parents – I felt completely alone.*'

Outcome: What would help your sad part settle? What does it need? What would it see as a good outcome to the argument?

_____

_____

Jasper's answer – '*To stop feeling so alone – to feel connected and liked by Janet.*'

Once you completed the above, see if you can gently come out of the 'skin' of your anxious part, and let that ease away. Take a few slower breaths, allowing your body to slow down. Now, see if you can put all the selves together by taking a moment to write down the answers you made in each of the above steps in Worksheet 23.1.

Worksheet 23.1: Multiple self exercise

Angry self	Sad self
Thoughts	Thoughts
Body	Body
Behaviour	Behaviour
Memory	Memory
Outcome	Outcome
Anxious self	**Compassionate self**
Thoughts	Thoughts
Body	Body
Behaviour	Behaviour
Memory	Memory
Outcome	Outcome

Self-reflection: It can be helpful to reflect on what you've learnt so far. What did you learn about the different parts of you in response to the same situation (the argument)?

_____

_____

_____

Did you find one 'part' easier to get into or think about than another? What do you make of that? Is that something that you recognise in other aspects of your life?

_____

_____

_____

Was there a part that was more difficult to connect with? What do you make of that? Is that something you recognise in other areas of your life?

_____

_____

A common response is to recognise that these three different parts (anger, anxiety, sadness) have very different ways of looking at, thinking and feeling about the same situation, and differ with regards to what they want and need. They also tend to connect to separate memories. Moreover, the way the different parts feel, and respond (and what they want) can conflict, and drive you in opposite directions (e.g. to angrily lash out or anxiously run away). This is an important reflection, as it can help us appreciate what our minds are up against, and the difficulties this can cause us. And whilst this is not our fault, having this insight can motivate us to learn how to be with all these different selves, and respond in ways that are helpful (we will return to this later in the chapter).

In our experience (both personally, and as therapists), it's also common that people find one of the 'selves' 'easier' to connect with and think from, and (at least) one that is more difficult to connect with. If that was the case for you, this is an important insight in itself, as it may help you to understand why you tend to respond in a typical way when arguments or conflict arise. This can also give us a clue as to what you might need your compassionate self to help you with. For example, your compassionate self might help you moderate or keep in balance the part of you that you most readily get drawn into (e.g. anger), and give space/ allow, support and strengthen the parts of you that you find difficult to connect with (e.g. sadness).

Box 23.1: Some tips to help with our multiple selves

Tips – to help with our multiple selves

- Allow yourself time to move into each 'part' – it sometimes takes a little while to find our way 'in' to each of these emotions, and it is often difficult if we feel rushed.

- Keep an eye on 'leakage'. This is when we are with one part of us (e.g. anxious) and another part of us (e.g. angry) 'spills in', making us feel and think differently. So for example, whilst describing what the anxious self would like to do in an argument we find that we have written down 'punch the idiot in the face'. It's unlikely that an anxious part of us would respond in this aggressive and violent way, and this is perhaps more indicative that we are connected with our angry self instead. If this is the case, spend some time to slow yourself down with your breathing rhythm, and then a little longer to connect with an anxious part of you. This leakage is understandable if some emotional selves are easier to connect with than others, as we suggested above.

- Try not to worry if you find one or more of these parts difficult to connect with. Most people find one part (if not more than one) more difficult than others to connect with or express. If this happens, take a little longer to try and shift into that self. Try to think about what that part (angry, anxious or sad) would say, or want to do, given the argument. Try not to get caught up in 'But I didn't feel like that during the argument'. This exercise is about exploring 'as if' scenarios, helping you to learn about your emotions (what each one thinks, wants to do and so forth), and recognising how these different parts of us can get caught up in conflicts that add to our struggles. So even if you weren't angry/anxious/sad in the argument, imagine how this part would have reacted/would like to react.

- Don't feel restricted to just these parts. You may want to do this exercise but have other parts present, such as shamed, guilty, proud, jealous, competitive, caring and so forth.

Step 4: How do the different parts relate to each other?

To deepen your understanding of our different 'selves', it can be helpful to consider what they think and feel about each other, and how they relate to each other. This step might feel a little strange, but in our experience, it adds to a deeper understanding of why we can struggle, or feel blocked, in experiencing and expressing certain emotions. Take a look back on what you've written for your angry, anxious and sad part above. Familiarise yourself again with how they see and feel about the argument, and their general outlook. Then see if you can answer the following questions:

How does the angry part think and feel about the anxious part?

_____

_____

How does the anxious part think and feel about the angry part?

_____

_____

How does the angry part think and feel about the sad part?

_____

_____

How does the sad part think and feel about the angry part?

_____

_____

How does the anxious part think and feel about the sad part?

_____

_____

How does the sad part think and feel about the anxious part?

_____

_____

Self-reflection: So, what was that like? What have you learnt about the interrelations between these different parts of you?

_____

_____

_____

_____

One common reflection at this stage is that these parts of us don't necessarily get on very well, or sit alongside each other comfortably. This is partly because they think, feel and want to do different, often competing things – for example, whilst anger often wants us to challenge or approach someone, anxiety is urging us to move away or avoid. Whilst this is understandable, it might become tricky for us if one particular part is more easily triggered, or experienced than another, and it keeps running the show! We can also consider why or how some emotional reactions (or selves) are blocked, inhibited or absent. But what can we do when we are pushed and pulled in different directions, really? Well, it might not surprise you that it can be helpful to connect with a part of us that can allow, listen to and help all different selves, and mediate between them. This, of course, would be *our compassionate self.*

Step 5: Bringing compassion to the situation

It is important at this stage to try and engage with our compassionate self in order to bring a different, more helpful, perspective to this situation. In these next sections, we are going to see how your compassionate self may help with bringing a perspective to the situation as a whole, but also in working with the different 'parts' (anger, anxiety, sadness) we looked at earlier.

As we have seen, depending on which part of us is viewing a situation, we are likely to think, feel and want to behave in quite different ways. Knowing this, if we engage our compassionate self, we are likely to approach the same situation with qualities of caring motivation, wisdom and strength, and a more balanced perspective. By engaging our compassionate self we can respond to situations in a way that is kinder, wiser and more courageous. To help you see this, have a go at the following exercise.

Exercise 1: Bringing Compassion to the Situation

Engage in your soothing rhythm breathing and friendly facial expression (see pages 122–28). Allow your breathing to slow a little, and gently rest your attention in the flow of breathing in, and breathing out. Bring to mind the qualities of your compassionate self – caring-commitment, wisdom and strength. When you feel ready, go through the following steps, answering from the perspective of your compassionate self.

Thoughts: What thoughts does your compassionate self have about the argument? What understanding or wisdom does it have about what happened?

_____

_____

Body: Where in your body do you feel the sense of strength, caring-commitment and wisdom of your compassionate self?

_____

Behaviour: If your compassionate self was in control, what would it want to do, given the situation (e.g. find a way to discuss the issue, rather than argue; help repair any damage caused; find a way to be assertive)?

_____

_____

Memories: Holding in mind your compassionate self, what memories come to mind?

_____

_____

Outcome: For your compassionate self, what would it see as a good outcome of this argument?

_____

_____

Self-reflection: What was seeing the argument from the compassionate self's perspective like? Did you notice any differences in comparison to the other parts?

_____

_____

Often people find that by embodying the compassionate self we can begin to look at, understand and respond to situations (in this case, an argument) in a very different way to the angry, anxious or sad part of ourselves. Given this, we may learn over time to consciously use our compassionate self to approach and work with our difficulties in life.

Step 6: Compassion for my different 'selves'

In this next stage, we are going to look at how our compassionate self can work in more detail with the individual parts – the angry, anxious and sad self. This is to help each part to feel heard and understood, whilst lessening the grip that a particular self might have on us, and bringing more balance and harmony between our different selves. For example, if our angry self takes over completely, this might result in a big fight, horrible things being said, and further unintended, but negative, consequences in the future. By using our compassionate self, we may find a way to tolerate and guide our angry part (or any other 'part' for that matter) so that it can play a useful role for us, but not at the expense of us, and our relationships.

We will go through this exercise in steps, taking each 'self' one at a time.

Compassion for My Angry Self

We all experience moments of anger but it can be helpful if we can find a way to understand and guide this part of us.

Exercise 2: Compassion for your angry self

Spend some time connecting with the soothing rhythm of your breathing (see pages 124–28). When you feel ready, bring to mind some of the qualities of compassion (caring-motivation, strength, wisdom). Once you feel connected with your compassionate self, bring to mind the angry part of you in the argument above.

What does your compassionate self want to say to the angry part of you? What does it understand about your angry part's reaction? What would your compassionate self suggest as helpful for the angry part? Is there something that it would like to do to help the angry self?

_____

_____

_____

_____

_____

_____

Jasper's answer – 'It's understandable that you're feeling angry about what happened, and the situation could have been very serious for the company. But the customer has agreed to meet next week, and you can speak to Janet about how she can learn from this and reduce the likelihood of this type of mistake happening in the future.'

Compassion for the anxious part of me

In this next exercise we want to turn the focus of your compassionate mind to the anxious self in the argument. Just as with anger, in Chapter 3 we learnt that anxiety evolved to help us pay attention to potential threats, and motivates us to move away, or flee as a way of keeping us safe. Let's see if we can use our compassionate self to understand and guide your anxious self in this situation.

Exercise 3: Compassion for Our Anxious Self

Engage in your soothing rhythm breathing (see pages 124–28), and slowly connect with the qualities of your compassionate self – caring-commitment, wisdom and strength. When you feel connected to this part of you, read through the questions below, making a few notes as you go.

What does your compassionate self want to say to the anxious part of you? What does it understand about the reactions of the anxious part, given the argument? Given its wisdom and caring-commitment, what would the compassionate self want to do for your anxious part? How would it like to help or support it?

_____

_____

_____

_____

_____

Jasper's answer – 'I can see why you feel like this; so much hard work has gone into the business, and so much depends on it, like the mortgage. I can also see that given your experience as a child, setbacks are likely to cause a lot of anxiety, and why it feels like running away will be easier. Although you're feeling anxious, I'm here to help out with this; if we take our time to look through the coming orders, we can organise a way of covering the shortfall. And I'll also be here to keep a lookout for problems like this in the future.'

Compassion for the sad part of me

Sadness can play an important role in signalling distress, often related to the experience of loss, and need for connection and support. However, for some of us, our sadness may not have been met with care or support from others, and feeling sad can be very difficult. Let's see what your compassionate self can do to understand and support your sad part.

Exercise 4: Compassion for Our Sad Self

Engage in your soothing rhythm breathing (see pages 124–28), and begin to connect with the attributes of your ideal compassionate self – caring-commitment, wisdom and strength. When you feel ready, from the perspective of your compassionate self, consider the following questions:

What does your compassionate self want to say to your sad self? What does your compassionate self understand about the reactions of your sad self, given the situation? What would your compassionate self like to do to support and help the sad part of you?

_____

_____

_____

_____

Jasper's answer – 'It's really understandable that you feel concerned and sad about potentially losing your friendship with Janet; she's been a great employee, and an even better friend. Although you're worried she'll end your friendship, remember that you've had fallouts with her before, and you've always found a way to repair things and get close again. I'm here to support you with all this – you're not alone.'

Self-reflection: What was this final part of the exercise like? What was it like to bring your compassionate self to relate to your angry, anxious and sad parts?

_____

_____

_____

_____

Summary

We often find that over time using the compassionate self may provide a helpful way to work with the common parts of us that turn up and influence how we respond to different (and difficult) situations we encounter in life. We can begin to learn that these parts often have important and useful things to say, and reasons for being there – but sometimes they need support and guidance and need to be heard. See if you can continue to practise this exercise in your day-to-day life. You may choose to use arguments as examples to explore your different parts, but our different selves show up rather commonly in many situations in life, such as:

- Making difficult decisions, when a part of us can feel one thing, and another part another.

- An important event – for example, attending an interview.

- A difficult encounter with someone, where the main experience may be being treated unfairly.

- Disappointments – for example, in relationships, or failing at, or losing, something that's important to us.

Remember when we are learning a new skill we need to build ourselves up gradually, as it can take a while to approach our life in this way. We would not learn to swim by diving from a boat into turbulent waters, we would start in the shallow end of a swimming pool!

Chapter summary

In this chapter we've explored the concept of our 'multiple selves' by focusing on how we can have different emotional experiences, and responses about the same incident, depending on which emotional part of us is guiding our thinking and behaviour.

What we have learnt together	My personal reflections on the chapter
1. We have 'multiple' selves – different parts of us that feel and react to a situation in quite different ways. 2. Some of us will find it easier to experience certain 'selves' (e.g. angry or anxious), and harder to experience others. This partly depends on our earlier experiences of learning. 3. Our compassionate self may be able to take a different and more helpful perspective to a given situation. 4. Our compassionate self may be helpful in understanding, supporting and guiding our other emotional selves.	

24 Working with common difficulties – Bringing our compassionate mind to shame and self-criticism

'Everyone is a moon, and has a dark side which he never shows to anybody.'

– *Mark Twain*

In the previous chapter we explored the idea that we are full of multiple parts, and how these can operate like subpersonalities. We also learned that some of us can get locked in a particular 'self' (e.g. anger or anxiety) that can cause us problems. One common and distressing experience is when we get caught in shame-based self-criticism. We are going to spend some time in this chapter reflecting on these experiences, how, and why we have them, and consider how our compassionate mind can help us address the difficulties that might arise as a result of them.

Understanding shame

We have all experienced shame in one form or another. Shame is a social emotion in which we feel that other people hold us in a negative light, and we feel that we are inadequate, inferior or defective in some way. Like any emotion, it can affect the way we think, pay attention, and behave. The origins of the word 'shame' are thought to come from an old word that means 'to cover'. Take a moment to think about this. When you felt ashamed about something, what was the urge in your body? What did you want to do? A common response is to hide, become smaller, or want to disappear or 'cover up' – to conceal the thing we feel ashamed about. The phrase 'hang your head in shame' gives an indication of the body posture that goes with shame.

Shame often pulls our attention towards what we feel ashamed about, or creates an urge to move ourselves away from this. This could be through avoidance, as well as by using distraction, or 'blocking' the experience (for example, by trying to focus on other things and suppress the shameful thoughts, or working relentlessly, drinking alcohol or using drugs, so as not to think and feel). Shame often blends with the emotions of the threat system – anxiety, anger and sometimes disgust – and many people describe it as one of the most unpleasant emotions to experience. In terms of our thinking, shame often comes with a self-critical, self-blaming or self-denigrating set of thoughts about ourselves, or what others think about us.

Why do we experience shame?

All of us will experience shame at some stage in our lives. To get to the heart of why this is the case, it may be helpful to consider what life would be like if we had *no* shame at all. So, take a moment to think about a *shameless person*, someone who has a complete inability to experience shame. How might this person relate to other people, and act? What would they be willing to do? What would they not be willing to do? Would you feel like getting emotionally close to this person, becoming friends with them?

For most people, the idea of being emotionally close to a shameless person is not very attractive – they are not the type of person we would feel comfortable being around, or indeed opening up to. So, can shame be desirable or useful to an extent? In fact, the function of shame is to signal to our threat system to pay attention to important social cues, tracking how our actions are impacting upon other people, and shaping us to act and behave in ways that fit with social rules and norms.

Shame operates in this way for some important reasons. Many thousands of years ago, our ancestors lived in environments that were tough. Food was scarce, the elements and weather harsh, and there were animals that could hurt or kill them. Within this context, our ancestors survived because they were part of a group. Group members protected each other from various dangers, hunted together, and shared food and shelter amongst themselves. However, consider what might happen if a group member did something that was harmful to another member, or didn't contribute to bringing in resources, or ate all the food. One punishment – particularly if the behaviour was very bad – would have been being excluded and ostracised from the group. This would mean having to deal with life's difficulties and dangers on one's own, and most likely, death would follow. The experience of shame has thus evolved to help us track how we exist in the minds of others and to avoid rejection, segregation, and ultimately death. Interestingly, when we connect about shame we are often concerned with others' negative judgements of us, being disliked, and not wanted. So, shame can be understood as a powerful echo from our past, and although unpleasant when experienced, it is tied to the threat system and has some important protective functions, directing us to pay attention to our behaviour and actions, and how we are 'living in the minds of others'. The fear that humans have of rejection, and importance of this in shame, means that shame is not an emotion that is easy to ignore. If shame is experienced in a relatively short time period, and at a level (intensity or power) that is tolerable, it can actually have a useful impact on shaping pro-social behaviour that is consistent with social norms and expectations. However, prolonged, all-pervasive and intense experiences of shame can result in a lot of internal distress, and this can inhibit pro-social behaviour.

The shame that disconnects

When shame is activated at a high level of intensity and over a prolonged period of time, it may serve as a block to the soothing-affiliative system. Let's take a moment to think about this. Imagine that you have a sense of deep shame about yourself – maybe that there is something about you that you believe is bad, ugly or flawed in some way. Imagine that you also think that your friends, family or colleagues hold these thoughts about you as well. Given that shame often urges us to want to conceal or hide in some way, it is likely that if you act on this urge (e.g. by socially withdrawing) this would disconnect you from people. It is true that, when we feel very ashamed, we typically do not feel open to the kindness, care or compassion of others, and find it difficult to have any self-compassion around these experiences. Moreover, if we distance ourselves from others, this tends not to help to resolve the feeling of shame, but, on the contrary, often exacerbates it. As we explored in Chapter 1, our new brain competencies for imagination, worry and rumination mean that we create threat-based (or shame-based, in this case) 'loops in the mind' in the absence of a real physical or social threat (see page 10). In other words, when we imagine others thinking badly of us or rejecting us (new brain), we experience this as 'real' and feel ashamed (old brain threat emotion). We then socially withdraw to protect ourselves (old brain fleeing behaviour), which leaves us with a profound sense of loneliness, which in turn directs our thinking and attention in a threat-focused (negative) way, and so on.

Compassion: An antidote for shame?

Given that shame is linked to the threat system and commonly blocks our connection to others (the soothing-affiliative system), it may be that compassion can play an important role in managing this experience. There are a number of steps to support this process.

1. Bring to mind something that you feel ashamed about. This might be something about yourself (for example, something to do with your body or personality), something that's happened in the past (e.g. a sense of having failed at something), or maybe something that you're struggling with now (such as a relationship, or your role at work). If it helps, make a few short notes below about why this is difficult.

    _____

    _____

    _____

2. Spend a few minutes connecting with your compassionate self. See if you can find the posture, breathing rhythm, and facial expression that facilitates this, and connecting with the qualities of wisdom, strength and commitment.

3. When you feel ready, see if you can use this compassionate part to look towards the shame you're experiencing. To start with, just see if you are able to tolerate this feeling. It might help here to really focus on the strength, groundedness and commitment (to be caring of yourself) of your compassionate self.

4. It might be helpful to bring the wisdom of your compassionate mind. Given what we've discussed above about the nature, origin and function of shame, you may be able to 'name' this. See if you can recognise how shame is a powerful feeling that human beings experience, and one that has evolved for our survival, and how it arrives with certain fears (e.g. rejection).

It can be useful to consider what your compassionate self may want to say to the part of you that feels ashamed, in a way that is caring, wise and encouraging. Maybe you could write a compassionate letter about this shame related difficulty (see Chapter 22 for a guide), complete a Compassionate Thought Form about this (Chapter 19). Take your time with this and give your compassionate self enough space to provide help and support.

Self-reflection: What was it like to try and bring compassion to your experience of shame? Did you notice any difference, or change in the feeling?

_____

_____

_____

_____

As we begin to bring our compassionate mind to our sense of shame, sometimes we can notice that the shame loses a bit of its ferocity and stickiness. Through the strength of our compassionate self, over time we can learn that we can tolerate the feeling and have the courage to work through it. The wisdom of our compassionate mind can help us appreciate that it's not our fault that we feel like this, and to understand that shame has evolved for a survival reason (to protect us from being ostracised, and dying alone) and that it's linked to our fears of rejection, which our personal experiences may have also left us sensitive to. The commitment and care of our compassionate self can support us in resisting what shame is urging us to do, and can help us to find a way to move towards more helpful solutions.

From shame to self-criticism: Understanding our self-critic

In Compassionate Mind Training (CMT), we separate one aspect of shame that focuses on what other people think of us (known as external shame, e.g. 'He must think I'm such a pathetic loser' and 'She'll always see me as weak for responding like that), from the shame that focuses on our own thoughts and feelings about ourselves. This type of shame – known as 'internal shame' – often comes with self-criticism, self-attack or even self-hatred. In many countries, particularly in the West, self-criticism is exceptionally common, sits at the heart of people's unhappiness and distress, and can keep us locked into our threat systems. In the remainder of this chapter, we're going to explore self-criticism in more detail, and learn how the skills you developed earlier can be combatted with wisdom, strength and commitment. It can be helpful to recognise that self-criticism can take on many different guises. Here, we're going to spend some time exploring some of the attributes of self-criticism, such as its focus, content, form, 'appearance' and emotional experiences that go with it, and its origins. To help us think about self-criticism, we will introduce Rashinda's story and, later on, use this to illustrate the different facets of shame.

Example: Rashinda was a young woman studying at university. She came to therapy describing how she was finding it difficult to concentrate on her studies, or take pleasure in social activities. She described frequently criticising herself, either for not getting 'perfect' marks in her essays, or for not being attractive enough, particularly in comparison with some of her friends. Rashinda described having a sense that she was inadequate, not good enough and inferior to others. She felt that her self-criticism was important because it urged her on to try harder and become more successful.

Rashinda described how her early life had been 'good', but that her father had been a tough disciplinarian. Although she knew he loved her, she recalled that growing up, he was always telling her 'You should be doing better' and 'You must improve, this is not good enough'. She had a particularly vivid memory of returning home feeling excited to have achieved 90 per cent in a test, only for her father to react with disappointment and focus on why she hadn't got 100 per cent.

We will come back to Rashida's experience shortly, but before we do, let's look at some of the attributes of self-criticism, one by one.

Focus: Our self-criticism can focus on, or be directed to, a broad range of things. Some of us are critical of our general appearance (e.g. 'I'm so ugly') or about particular characteristics (e.g. 'My nose us too big', 'My thighs too fat', 'I'm not tall enough'). Our self-criticism can be focused on aspects of our personality (e.g. 'I'm so boring'), or our abilities, such as our intelligence (e.g. 'I'm such a stupid, thick idiot'). Sometimes our self-criticism is directed to our mistakes (either current or past), or even to anticipated future mistakes (e.g. 'I'll mess up'). Often self-criticism involves a comparison with others, in a way that we feel more inferior and worse off (e.g. 'I'm not as intelligent/interesting/beautiful/successful as others').

Self-reflection: Spend a moment to think about your self-criticism. What does it tend to focus upon?

_____

_____

Rashinda's answer – 'My criticism focuses on my mistakes and failures, and times when I haven't achieved perfection. It also focuses on my appearance – particularly my face and my stomach.'

Content: Sometimes it can be helpful to notice the content of our self-criticism; that is, the actual words that we use (internally or out loud) when we are critical with ourselves. For example, a former client told one of us that their self-criticism tended to involve light-hearted content: 'You silly sausage!', which didn't cause them much distress. However, another client described something very different: 'You really messed that up, didn't you, you *stupid, pathetic* piece of shit!' As you might guess, the harsh language of this latter criticism can be far more distressing.

Self-reflection: Spend a moment thinking about the content of your self-criticism. Are there certain types of words or phrases that are common?

_____

_____

_____

Rashinda's answer – 'It can be quite hostile. Things like: 'You stupid piece of shit!' or 'Your face is so ugly and big'.

Form: Whilst the content of our self-criticism can be important, research studies have shown the *form* it takes is also important. In fact, research by Professor Paul Gilbert and one of us (CI) found that self-criticism can take at least two forms: one in which self-criticism is associated with feeling put-down and inadequate after failures and setbacks, and a more destructive, disgust-based response to setbacks that can include an aggressive desire to punish ourselves for this.

Self-reflection: Think about the type of self-criticism you have after a setback or failure. Does this take the form of feeling inadequate and not good enough, or of disgust or anger towards yourself?

_____

_____

Rashinda's answer – 'My self-criticism is mostly about me being inferior and inadequate, but I can see that sometimes it takes a more angry form when I really hate myself.'

Image and emotion: One helpful way of exploring the nature of our self-criticism is through the use of imagery. This can help us to get a physical perspective in our minds of what our self-criticism would look like, sound and feel like. This can help to move out of 'thinking about', and connect more with the felt experience of self-criticism.

To do this, find somewhere quiet where you won't be disturbed for five minutes. Close your eyes, and take some time to bring to mind the types of things you criticise yourself for. When you feel ready, try to imagine what your self-critic would look like if you could take it out of your head, and see it in front of you. Pay attention to its facial expression (if it has a face), its size, voice tone (if it has a voice), its movements, and what emotions it is directing towards you.

Self-reflection: What does your self-critic look like (size, facial expression, voice tone)?

_____

_____

_____

_____

What emotion is it directing to you? How do you feel in the presence of your self-critic, particularly given the emotion it is directing to you?

_____

_____

Rashinda's answer – 'I can picture my inner critic as a stern, middle-aged man. He is tall, he has a stick that he is waving about, and he has a mean look on his face and is shaking his head disapprovingly. He is angry and aggressive. I feel anxious, tense and small in comparison.'

Self-reflection: What have you learnt from imagining your self-critic?

Rashinda's answer – 'My self-critic is very angry and aggressive and it leaves me feeling anxious, and on edge. It reminds me of my father, in an exaggerated way. I didn't realise my self-criticism was so powerful, or full or anger.'

Function: Another way of learning about your self-critic is thinking about the function that it has, or plays, for you. One way to explore the function(s) of your self-critic is to use functional analysis. This is a method of looking at, or discovering, what a particular thought, behaviour, response or emotion serves; what its purpose (or function) is. One way that we can discover the function of our self-critic is to ask ourselves:

Self-reflection: What would my fear be if, somehow, I could never be self-critical again? Would I lose anything, or would there be any costs to this for me?

Rashinda's answer – 'I fear that my standards would drop and I will not be good enough – and if this happens, people will not want to be around me, and I'll be on my own.'

Box 24.1: Common functions of self-criticism

Often, although not always, people notice that when they start imagining giving up their self-criticism, there will be an unpleasant, and painful consequence, which is usually related to the activation of the threat system. Let's take a look at three different examples of this:

- Leroy, a hardworking but struggling journalist, felt concerned that, without his self-critic, he would make mistakes and, ultimately, be unsuccessful and unhappy.

- Claire, a kind and caring nurse struggling with burnout, was worried that without her self-critic, she would become arrogant and 'too big for her boots', and as a consequence, people wouldn't like her.

- Clive, a 50-year-old business manager who came to therapy for problems with assertiveness, realised that he feared that, without his self-critic, he would become very angry with people in his life. His concern was that without his self-critic keeping a lid on his anger, he could become a 'tyrant' and end up hurting and pushing people away.

To help you understand a little more about this, let's take a look at some of the questions below, which have been taken from the Functions of Self-Criticism Scale, which was developed by Paul Gilbert and colleagues. The questionnaire measures two different functions of self-criticism: to self-correct/improve, and to persecute and punish. In the chart below we have given some examples of the two functions of self-criticism.

I get critical and angry with myself:	Yes	No
To make sure I keep up my standards.		
To stop myself being happy.		
To show I care about my mistakes.		
Because if I punish myself I feel better.		
To stop me being lazy.		
To harm part of myself.		
To keep myself in check.		
To punish myself for my mistakes.		
To stop me getting overconfident.		

To stop me being angry with others.		
To make me concentrate.		
To gain reassurance from others.		
To prevent future embarrassments.		

Self-reflection: Having completed the above, what do you think might be the function, or role, your self-criticism plays for you?

_____

_____

Origin: Where did your self-critic come from?

We can try and understand our self-critic by considering where it came from, and how it developed. There can be a number of origins, or sources of self-criticism:

1. Relational experiences: The types of relationships we had (or have) may play a role in shaping our self-criticism. For example, if we had relationships with people who were hostile, critical, rejecting or bullying, we may have learned to speak to ourselves in similar ways by directing criticism and hostility to ourselves.

2. Trauma: Self-criticism could be a result of traumatic life experiences. There is considerable research evidence that individuals who have experienced trauma, especially of an interpersonal nature, such as domestic violence, child abuse, or bullying, are more likely to have symptoms of shame and self-criticism.

3. Failure: Key setbacks and failures (e.g. being made redundant; disappointing exam results) can sometimes be a trigger for self-critical thoughts. For some people, public setbacks, particularly those that involve a sense of shame (being seen as 'lesser' by others), can trigger self-criticism.

4. Media: There is considerable evidence that messages from the media (adverts, movies and magazines), which portray ideas about how we should look (e.g. our body shape, facial features, clothing, etc.) and what type of possessions we should have (e.g. phones, bags, cars) can influence our sense of self (our self-esteem) and contribute to a sense of feeling 'lesser than', or inferior,

to others. We tend to engage in social comparisons, seeing ourselves as less competent, less attractive, less well-off, and ultimately less 'worthy' than other people, and criticise ourselves.

Self-reflection: Think about your self-criticism. Do you have a sense of its origin? What has influenced its development?

_____

_____

_____

Bringing your compassionate mind to help your self-critic

Hopefully the exercises in this chapter will have helped you familiarise yourself with your self-critic, and its nature. Often, this greater understanding can be helpful in and of itself. Of course, turning towards this inner, painful experience can be challenging, and may leave us feeling rather sensitive. It is here where compassion becomes important. We are going to spend the rest of this chapter considering how we can bring our compassionate mind to engage with our self-critical part in order to lessen its (at times) unhelpful and painful impact on us. We will do this in a number of steps:

Step 1: Being aware of self-criticism

Initially, it can be helpful for us to become more mindfully aware of our self-criticism. Becoming more aware of your self-criticism will help you connect to the first psychology of compassion: being sensitive to your own distress and suffering. In our therapeutic work, we have often noticed that on asking clients about their self-critic, some respond: 'I'm not very self-critical', or 'I don't criticise myself very often'. However, when people are asked to tune into their inner experience in a mindful way (paying attention to its form, function, focus, and emotions involved), they often realise just how powerful and pervasive their self-criticism is. In fact, a client told us: 'My self-criticism is like breathing to me, I don't even notice it most of the time. It's only when I started to pay attention to it that I began to notice what it was really like.'

It can be helpful to use Worksheet 24.1 on page 335 to monitor and record the frequency and form of your self-criticism over a period of time. First, let's return to Rashinda and look at her diary as an example.

Self-criticism log – Rashinda

Date	What was I doing? What triggered my self-criticism?	What did I say to myself? What was the focus of my self-criticism?	Why was I critical? What was my criticism trying to do?	How did being self-critical leave me feeling?
24 July	Filling in an application form and having to put my A-level results down.	I told myself I was stupid and that my friends were more intelligent than I am.	I was critical because I want to keep my standards up, so that other people won't criticise me.	I felt sad, useless and inferior.
4 August	I look fat in this dress.	I compared myself with my sister – I'm less attractive, less popular and less respected.	Being self-critical reminds me to work on my diet and keep to my fitness regime.	I'm disappointed with myself for not being able to look as good as others – I'm a loser in life.
22 August	Thinking about my exam results.	I told myself that I am not smart enough. I should have done better.	So I don't let myself down again and to remind myself to try harder in future.	Frustrated and sad.

Worksheet 24.1: Self-criticism Log

Date	What was I doing? What triggered my self-criticism?	What did I say to myself? What was the focus of my self-criticism?	Why was I critical? What was my criticism trying to do?	How did being self-critical leave me feeling?

Step 2: Listening to and validating our self-criticism

As we explored previously, the idea of losing our self-criticism can trigger our threat system. We often fear that without our self-critic, we might become selfish, arrogant, lazy, angry, or uncaring. If we can see this fear as an understandable threat response, we can bring our compassionate mind to understand this fear, validate it, and try to work with this in the same way we might try to help an anxious part of us. Our compassionate mind may be able to recognise that our self-criticism can have an important role in signalling to us to be aware of a potential threat. Equally, our compassionate mind would be able to see how this inner critic can leave us feeling low in mood, lacking in confidence, and even depressed. One way that we can think about this experientially is the following:

Example: Two teachers

Imagine that a child you really care about is struggling with maths at school. This could be your own child, a relative, or a friend's child. Imagine that they find it very hard to understand different maths concepts, and often feel stressed and ashamed in class. Unfortunately, things feel even worse for them, as the other students seem to be taking it all in easily. Given this situation, how would you feel if the image of your self-critic – the one you identified in the exercise on page 335 – was the teacher of this child who was struggling?

Self-reflection: How do you imagine this would leave the child feeling? Would this critic be helpful in enabling the child to deal with this challenge, and improve at maths?

_____

_____

_____

_____

It's likely that most of you don't like the idea of your critic being the teacher of a child who is struggling; somehow intuitively this doesn't feel right. But isn't it interesting that whilst we wouldn't want our critic let out onto others, we are threatened by the idea of letting this go from our side?

We can take the above example a step further. What sort of teacher would you like this child to have? Think about the type of qualities you would like them to carry in order to be helpful, and make a note of them below:

_____

_____

_____

Common attributes that people report here include patience, encouragement, compassion, kindness, support, warmth and persistence – qualities that are often closely aligned with those of the compassionate self or compassionate other. Why is this important? Well, in some ways, sometimes our compassionate self and our self-critic are similar in that neither wants to see us make mistakes, struggle, become lazy, arrogant or selfish, or be alone. The self-critic does this through fear and threat, whereas the compassionate self does this through understanding, encouragement and care.

Step 3: Compassionate engagement of the self-critic

This next phase involves using your compassionate mind to engage with your self-critic. We are going to guide you using the skills that you've developed throughout this book.

Exercise 1: Using Our Compassionate Self to Work with Self-criticism

To start with, find a place to sit in an upright but comfortable position. Take your time to bring your awareness into the here and now, connecting with your soothing rhythm breathing (see pages 124–28). After a minute or two, bring to mind the qualities of your compassionate self – wisdom, strength and commitment. Take a few moments to see if you can step into the shoes of your compassionate self and connect with your compassionate facial expression, voice tone and body posture. When you feel connected with this part of you, imagine that you can see the image of your self-critic in front of you – the image that you developed earlier in this chapter. Gently direct the qualities of your compassionate self towards your self-critic. See if you can use the following as a guide:

Wisdom and understanding – Upon looking at your self-critic, what can you understand about it? What is it trying to do for you? What is its function? Can you see what emotions sit behind the critic, or what fears it has about you, or the world around you? Your compassionate self may have some empathy and understanding of what has made the critic act in this way. See if you can direct compassion to both the critic, and also the reasons for why it directs criticism to you.

Strength and confidence – Sometimes in the face of our self-critics, we can begin to feel threatened, anxious or overwhelmed ourselves. To help with this, focus on the strength and groundedness of your compassionate self. Notice your upright body posture and ability to tolerate difficulties. If you do feel a bit overwhelmed, you might imagine taking a couple of steps back from the image of your self-critic, tuning back into your soothing rhythm breathing, and re-connecting with the strength of your compassionate self.

Caring-motivation – Holding onto your desire to be caring and supportive, how might you communicate this to your self-critic? As your compassionate self, what would you like to say or do for your self-critic? Is there a way you could help the critic with his concerns, but maybe in a more caring and wise way?

Notice what happens to the image or your self-critic as you direct compassion to it from your compassionate self.

When you feel ready, allow the image of your self-critic to fade from your mind. Tune back into your soothing rhythm breathing for a few moments. When you feel ready, bring yourself back into the room.

Self-reflection: What was this exercise like for you? Was your compassionate self able to offer some support or understanding for your critic?

_____

_____

_____

_____

Step 4: Changing shame-based self-criticism to compassionate self-correction

As we've been exploring above, rather than trying to take away our self-critic (which tends to trigger the threat system as it is often trying to protect us), we are trying to channel our self-criticism in such a way that some of its helpful aims can remain, but in a spirit of warmth, encouragement, and care. Often we refer to this as *compassionate self-correction*. The idea here is that our compassionate self helps us turn towards our difficulties, and motivates us to take responsibility to work on them, in a way that is encouraging and supportive and wise. Have a look at the table below – here, we can consider some of the differences between self-criticism and self-correction.

Shame-based self-criticism	Self-correction
Shame-based self-criticism is associated with threat-based emotions (fear, shame and anger) and relates to:	Self-correction involves a desire to do our best, to be open to our limitations in and wanting to learn and improve skills and focuses on:
• A wish to punish and condemn • Fear of failure • Blaming and shaming • Feelings of disappointment with oneself, anger and frustration • Avoidance of situations • Social comparisons, where the self is inferior, and judged against specific standards.	• A desire to improve • Growth and enhancement • Giving support, encouragement and kindness • Acknowledges what goes well and considers areas for development • Appreciation and acceptance of the self as whole.

Hopefully you'll be able to see from the table above that self-compassion is not about being nice, or letting ourselves off the hook. We are instead talking about developing a compassionate coach, a compassionate-corrector that can help us to manage the difficulties in life with wisdom and strength. It can be helpful, when imagining directing compassion to your self-critic as your compassionate self, to point out to the critic that you also have your best interests at heart and want to help yourself flourish and be happy.

Self-reflection: Holding in mind the idea of compassionate self-correction, how could you apply this in your life? If you were to bring this perspective – rather than a purely shame-based self-critical one – to something that you were recently criticising yourself for, what would be the difference?

_____

_____

_____

_____

What is your intention for how you will compassionately react to setbacks, mistakes or failures in the future?

_____

_____

Chapter summary

In this chapter we have explored how shame and self-criticism can be common, yet difficult experiences for us, and how compassion may be a way to work with these experiences.

What we have learnt together	My personal reflections on the chapter
1. Shame is a common human experience that influences the way we think, feel and behave.	
2. Shame can be a potent disconnector to the care and compassion of other people, and blocks our capacity to be self-compassionate.	

3. Self-criticism can be linked to shame, and has multiple components, including what it focuses on, and what its function is.

4. We can use our compassionate mind to alleviate the pain associated with the experience of self-criticism. We can learn to understand and validate our self-critic, and find a way of moving towards compassionate self-correction, rather than shame based self-criticism.

25 Working with common difficulties – How to manage fears, blocks or resistances to compassion

'A journey of a thousand miles begins with a single step.'

– Chinese Proverb

As we've moved through this workbook, we've tried to highlight how compassion can play a powerful role in helping us to engage with, understand and find ways of alleviating distress. We are hoping that we have managed to convey how the compassionate approach to life, and its difficulties, can be beneficial to our emotional wellbeing and relationships. This of course does not mean that being compassionate or receiving compassion is easy and straightforward. In fact, for many of us, compassion often comes with challenges, as it can be a source of distress and anxiety. Before reading on, you may find it helpful to return to Chapter 7, where we looked at some of the specific fears, blocks and resistances to compassion (see pages 94–98). This chapter will explore some of the challenges in the experience of compassion, focusing on four common difficulties, along with some ideas for what we can do to manage these if they arise.

1. Compassion is a weakness or indulgence

If you think that compassion is inherently a weakness, indulgence or involves letting you (or others) off the hook, the process of cultivating your compassionate mind is likely to be quite difficult. These beliefs about compassion are quite common, and are sometimes shaped by our experiences in life. For example, if we have been raised in a family or have attended a school that voiced beliefs that compassion is self-focused, selfish and weak, it is likely that we may go on to hold similar beliefs, concerns or worries about it. We may also receive these same messages from our culture (e.g. magazines, newspapers, music and TV).

Let's consider some of the ways that we can work with such beliefs:

- It can be helpful to start by validating these concerns. It's understandable that we would find developing our skills in compassion difficult if we believe that in doing so, we would become a selfish, self-indulgent and weak person.

- It can also be useful to consider where this belief or concern may come from. If we've been exposed to or been taught that this is what other people feel compassion is, or leads to, it's not surprising that we may also share some of these beliefs.

- It can be useful to remind ourselves of the definition of compassion we are using in Compassionate Mind Training (CMT) – Compassion is the sensitivity to the suffering of self and others, with a commitment to relieve it. Based on this, we can see that, on the contrary to being a weakness or indulgence, compassion actually involves strength and courage to engage with pain and distress, and wisdom, dedication and motivation to reduce this pain, or what is causing it. Compassion is really about facing difficulties, rather than running away from them. Becoming aware and mindful of our negative beliefs about compassion, and the fears involved, can be a helpful first step in itself. This can help us stand back from these beliefs rather than react to them, recognising activation of our threat system and tolerating the discomfort this may bring.

- It can be useful to reflect on how you would respond if a close friend or loved one held the belief that being compassionate to themselves was a weakness or indulgence.

Self-reflection: How would you feel and think if someone you cared about held the view that showing compassion to themselves was weak? What would you say to them, if you were being caring and supportive? Do you see any discrepancy between your view about others having compassion for themselves and you being self-compassionate? If so, what can you learn from this that might help you in your journey towards developing your compassionate mind?

---

2. I don't deserve compassion

For some of us, the block to compassion is not related to a sense of weakness or indulgence. Rather, we might indeed see this as a positive experience other people deserve to have, but feel undeserving of it ourselves. There may be a number of ideas about how we can understand why this might be the case, and things we can do to support ourselves if we experience this type of block.

- Sometimes it can be helpful to reflect on when and how we learned that we didn't deserve compassion. Do you remember when you first thought you were undeserving of compassion? Did anyone (e.g. a family member or teacher) communicate this to you in some way? Sometimes recognising that our beliefs and fears about compassion, and sense of not deserving it, were shaped by certain experiences and/or relationships that were not of our choosing can be useful in bringing wisdom to this block. Once we are aware of this, we can begin to have compassion for those experiences that shaped our fears and threats about compassion.

- It may be helpful to consider which system is underneath this: is it your threat system that is reacting to the idea of you being non-deserving of compassion? If so, what is your fear here? Is there a concern or fear about having something that you feel hasn't been deserved? (And if so, can you reflect on what the concern may be here?) Where does this come from, and how true is it? Or is there an aspect of your drive system speaking here – that this, alongside your threat system – is suggesting that you can only experience compassion from others, and experience compassion for yourself, if you have achieved certain things in life? Do you feel that you have to earn compassion (from others or yourself) in some way? Sometimes, our sense of not deserving compassion emerges from our feeling or shame and self-critical thoughts. It may be worth reflecting on whether this is the case for you, and if so, it might be helpful to return to Chapter 24 to explore ideas about your self-criticism in more detail.

- If we can understand that this sense of non-deserving is linked to our threat or drive system, and perhaps past experiences we didn't choose, then we may try to have compassion for that instead. In other words, we can try to stay open to our difficulty with struggling to connect with compassion, bringing empathy and compassion to the reality of our struggle with this. Again, we might consider what small steps are here. For example, would it be possible, even if you don't feel you deserve compassion, to experiment with what happens if you do spend some time practising being more compassionate? Almost as though you are a sceptical scientist, unconvinced about the success of a particular experiment, but willing to try it and be guided by the results, rather than your initial belief.

Self-reflection: _____

_____

_____

3. Compassion is unfamiliar to me

Sometimes our difficulties with compassion are linked to how unfamiliar it is. Sadly, for some of us, we've had very few experiences of other people being a kind, caring and nurturing presence in our life, and instead, have often experienced others being threatening or shaming instead. Some of us may live in cultures, communities or even countries that promote and encourage other types of behaviour (e.g. competition) rather than compassion. There are a number of things that might be helpful here.

- Practice helps us to become more familiar. Just like learning a new language, sport or skill (e.g. a musical instrument), spending time practising compassion, even if we are not quite 'feeling' it in the beginning, is likely to help us to feel more comfortable and at ease with this experience.

- It could be helpful to start off with small steps – for example, engaging in one compassionate behaviour (or an act of kindness) each day, or practising one of the compassionate exercises (see Sections IV and V, pages 163–217) for a minute or two, each day.

- It can be useful to pay attention to the different forms compassion takes. For example, setting our intention to try and observe the compassion and care coming from others, this way familiarising ourselves with the experience, and stepping out of our threat system, where we spend most of our time.

4. Compassion triggers painful feelings in me

For some of us, compassion can evoke a painful experience, including feelings of anxiety, and anger. This could be associated with painful life experiences, such as being hurt by other people's words, or actions. The experience of compassion can also remind us of something or someone that we have lost, such as a pet, partner or family member, which may leave us feeling very sad, distressed and connected with grief. Compassion may also confront us with feelings of anger or sadness that we never had loving parents, family members or friends in our life. If you have any experiences like this, see if the guide below can support you:

- Small steps are often the key here – try not to rush or 'force' yourself to become more compassionate. As our colleague Dr Russell Kolts says, sometimes it's helpful to see how humans are like frozen shrimps! If you buy a packet of shrimps from your local supermarket, the instructions tell you not to force-thaw them in the microwave or under running water. Rather, you're advised to thaw them out slowly in the fridge. If you try to force-thaw them, they get all mushy and lose their shape, whereas defrosting them slowly allows them to retain their shape, and their taste. Dr Kolts' point here is that if we try to force ourselves to experience compassion, this can overwhelm us and make it harder to find a grounded position from which to engage with this work. This wisdom can thus support us to take this process slowly, patiently and in a step-by-step way, so as to maximise our chances of developing a strong and adaptive compassionate self.

You might also find it helpful to take a look at Box 25.1 below, which includes some general tips about how to manage fears, blocks and resistances to compassion.

Box 25.1: Tips – on how to manage fears, blocks and resistances to compassion

Tips – how to manage fears, blocks and resistances to compassion

- Start where you can – with small steps. For example, see if you can notice and stay open to moments of others being kind or caring to you (e.g. this could be a shop assistant or a colleague). The key is not to ignore the small, day-to-day examples of this (e.g. someone holding a door open for you, someone smiling and wishing you a nice day). Being aware of kind gestures, however small, can help your mind become familiar with this experience.

- Remember the three-system model, and see if you can notice when your threat system is coming on line. When you notice this, rather than judge the experience, see if you can return to your soothing breathing, compassionate colour or safe place image to help regulate the threat response, as a start.

- It could be helpful to remember the idea of 'old brain – new brain'. Are there any loops between the two that you can notice in understanding what is blocking your experience of compassion from (or to) others, or towards yourself? If this is the case, see if you can be mindful of these loops, and try to step back and refocus on your intention to remain open to signals of care as well as you can. If you notice a threat response emerging during this process – for example, anxiety or sadness – see if you can validate, and endure this experience, using your compassionate self.

• Finally, see if you can start by connecting with some compassion towards this struggle you're having (with compassion). This bringing compassion for our struggle with compassion might feel like a bit of a leap, but see if you can stick with it! See if you can stay sensitive and strong with respect to this understandable struggle without trying to push the discomfort away or get annoyed with it or yourself. This could be the very first step towards alleviating some of the struggle.

The compassionate ladder

A simple but helpful way to manage some of the difficulties in experiencing compassion is by using the metaphor of the 'compassionate ladder'. The idea is simple; when you stumble upon any blocks with some of the exercises, you can always move down the rungs of your compassionate ladder at your own pace, choosing to engage in exercises that you find easier to engage with but that also help you to manage your threat system. For example, if you find practising the 'ideal compassionate other' exercise tough, and that this has stirred up feelings of sadness and loss because the person who used to provide this compassion for you (your grandmother) passed away recently, you can perhaps move down the ladder to doing one of the compassionate mind training exercises that you feel might help to manage your distress and help you feel more grounded. For example, Louise had an experience very similar to this, and was able to move down her ladder from the compassionate other exercise, to the image of her 'safe place' imagery for a while. This, alongside her soothing breathing, helped her to feel more balanced and grounded, and helped to regulate her sadness and distress.

If you find 'safe place' imagery hard, then you can move a step down to practising soothing breathing, to calm your body and mind down, and feel secure in this before taking the next step. With consistent practice, over time you will gradually feel more secure and confident to move up the ladder again. Do your best not to come off the ladder completely, remembering that you can also return to your mindfulness exercises as a way of grounding yourself in the here and now.

Take a look at diagram 25.2 overleaf. Here, we've displayed the ladder in the steps that we've introduced the practices in this book, but in our experience each of us is likely to find one or another exercise in this book easier or harder than others. So it might be that the rungs of your 'ladder' are different to those illustrated in the diagram, and that you want to re-order how high up (harder, maybe more difficult or activating of threat system) and lower down (generally easier to connect with, practise and experience threat system regulation by doing).

Diagram 25.2: The Compassionate Ladder:
How to manage difficulties with CMT exercises

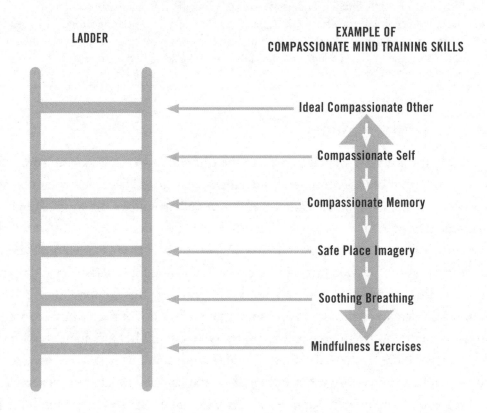

LADDER

EXAMPLE OF
COMPASSIONATE MIND TRAINING SKILLS

Ideal Compassionate Other

Compassionate Self

Compassionate Memory

Safe Place Imagery

Soothing Breathing

Mindfulness Exercises

Self-reflection: What would your 'ladder' look like? That is, would it be the same as above, or slightly different? Would it be helpful to draw out the rungs of your own ladder, based on the experiences you've had throughout doing the practices in this book? How could you hold in mind this idea of the compassionate ladder to help you manage any difficulties, blocks or fears that you're having with compassionate mind training exercises?

_____

_____

_____

_____

Chapter summary

In this chapter we have looked at how the experience of compassion can often be challenging, and how we can support ourselves with these challenges.

What we have learnt together	My personal reflections on the chapter
1. For some of us, experiencing compassion can be difficult. 2. Accepting that we have fears, blocks and resistances around compassion, in a non-judging or blaming way, is an important first step in moving forward. 3. We can use the 'rungs on a ladder' to face challenges with compassion in a patient, gradual and step-by-step way.	

SECTION VIII

LOOKING FORWARD:
Sustaining Our Compassionate Mind

In this final section of the workbook, we are going to focus on how we can help you to use the skills that you have developed in this book in the future.

As many of you will have experienced, it's one thing to go on a diet for a few days, or go to the gym for a week or two, but sustaining these changes can be laced with problems, pitfalls and setbacks. Our experience has been that it can be the same with developing your compassionate mind, and it can therefore be helpful to spend time considering ways to help work with this.

26 Looking forward – Sustaining our compassionate mind

'When you walk to the edge of all the light you have and take that first step into the darkness of the unknown, you must believe that one of two things will happen: There will be something solid for you to stand upon, or, you will be taught how to fly'.

– Patrick Overton, The Leaning Tree (1975)

We've covered a lot in this book together: Ideas about evolution, our tricky brains, the three-system emotion regulation model, and ideas about how your past and current relationships have shaped you. We've practised a variety of skills to help you develop your compassionate mind. These have included attention training and mindfulness, breathing work, imagery, shaping your thinking, and practising giving and receiving compassion. We have also considered how we can direct these insights and skills to common difficulties we struggle with, such as self-criticism, and difficult emotions. We hope that, through all this, you have been able to increase your understanding of yourself, and what causes you distress, and how your compassionate mind can support you in coping and dealing with this.

It may be helpful to use Worksheet 26:1 to reflect on what you've learnt and achieved whilst working through this book.

Worksheet 26:1: What I have Learnt and Achieved

What I've Learnt and Achieved

What I have learnt in this workbook:

_____

_____

_____

My achievements include:

_____

_____

_____

The challenges that I have faced and coped with are:

_____

_____

_____

I've coped with these difficulties by:

_____

_____

_____

Learning these skills, and cultivating a compassionate mind does not mean we will no longer experience setbacks, pain and suffering; this is an inevitable experience of the human condition.

As the old Chinese proverb goes: 'We can't stop the birds of sorrow flying above our head, but we can stop them building a nest in our hair.' In fact, the fostering of compassion is an on-going, life-long process, just as pain is an ever-present experience in life. In this chapter we will explore healthy, compassionate ways to deal with setbacks.

Intention for the future – sustaining our compassionate minds

Given your reflections on your achievements, progress and difficulties from working through the different sections of this book, it is important that you try to set an intention for how you are going to continue this journey in the future. Just as our bodies can become fit and strong if we regularly exercise but lose their condition and muscle strength if we stop, our compassionate minds can also lose their 'fitness' if we don't continue to cultivate and train them. Many people experience a variety of benefits when they practise the workbook's exercises regularly, and some of these benefits might last, even if they take a temporary break in their practice. However, over time the 'compassion muscles' begin to weaken and lose their strength in being able to help us.

We often say that a garden can grow in many ways, with grass, weeds, flowers and plants all vying for space. However, if you would like your garden to look a certain way, maybe to have a trimmed lawn, pruned plants and a flower-bed absent of weeds, you'll need to spend time and effort cultivating and tending it. Our minds are similar – they need continued effort and attention to grow in a way that will be helpful to us.

See if you can spend some time reflecting on what you will need to ensure that your compassionate mind continues to be nurtured and nourished. If you want, you can take a minute or two to connect with your compassionate self, its wisdom, strength and commitment, and see through its eyes.

Self-reflection: What would your compassionate self say in regard to maintaining your compassionate muscles, or garden?

_____

_____

_____

Personal practice diary

When working on developing your compassionate mind it might be helpful to create your own 'personal practice diary'. This may help you to track your progress and monitor changes, remind you of your achievements, and help you to notice and respond to any difficulties along your journey of compassion. Logging what you have practised and its impact on you can guide your journey, highlighting which skills are helpful, and what experiences you may want, or need, to work further on. This can also act as a 'compassionate coach', witnessing and supporting you in your journey. We have created a diary sheet below to support you in this process.

Worksheet 26.2: Compassionate Mind Practice Log

What have I found useful and would like to practise in the coming days, weeks and months?

What will help me keep up this practice?

What have I found helpful that I would like to practise when all is going well in my life?

_____

_____

_____

_____

What will help me keep up this practice?

_____

_____

_____

_____

What have I found helpful, and would like to practise when I am going through a tough time?

_____

_____

_____

_____

What will help me keep up this practice?

_____

_____

_____

_____

Developing a 'Compassionate Setback Plan'

As we mentioned earlier in this chapter, in our journey of developing our compassionate minds we might experience a number difficulties, setbacks and frustrations. One way of bringing compassion to these setbacks is by using a Compassionate Setback Plan (CSP). Developing a CSP involves spending time considering some of the challenges we might encounter in life, and more specifically in relation to cultivating and maintaining our compassionate minds. Although we cannot predict all of the setbacks we will encounter in life, the CSP can reflect on possible challenges and prepare us, by way of making a commitment to stay as caring, wise and strong of ourselves and others, in the face of them.

Of course, to develop your CSP it would be important to approach this task with a compassionate mind. So, before reflecting on Worksheet 26.3, spend a few moments connecting with your breathing rhythm and the qualities of your compassionate self – caring-commitment, wisdom and strength.

Worksheet 26.3: My setback plan

My setback plan
What situations might lead to a setback? (e.g. stress at work, starting a new relationship, financial problems)
What does your compassionate self say about possible setbacks in the future?

What would tell me that I'm getting caught in old patterns? What experiences (thoughts, behaviours, emotions, physical responses) could act as warning signs that I might be struggling?

_____

_____

_____

_____

_____

_____

How can my compassionate self help me to prepare for, or prevent these setbacks?

_____

_____

How can my compassionate self help me to work through and overcome these setbacks?

_____

_____

It can be helpful to have some of these ideas at hand and to keep them updated. What might be potential setbacks today may not be the same in a week, a month or even a year's time. Key, as ever, is to use the wisdom and caring motivation of your compassionate self to guide you with this. Sometimes people find it helpful to make a note of a few of the ideas from the CSP on a flashcard, or on their smartphone, so that it's easily accessible when needed.

Conclusion

'The finishing line is just the beginning of whole new race.' – *Teddy Ebersol*

So, as we come to the end of this workbook, and the end of our journey together, we'd both like to say 'well done' for getting here. Do remember we all experience setbacks, frustrations and struggles – this is part of life and what it means to be human. Rather than constantly trying to stop them happening or angrily fighting them, we can learn to try to deal with them as best we can, as they arise. This is self-compassion embodied. The key thing is to keep on nourishing and nurturing your compassionate self, to use it as a guide in moving forward, in the direction that you want.

So, going forward, all we would ask is that you continue to focus on being the version of you that is wise, strong and committed. We encourage you to continue to use your compassionate mind to help you face whatever difficulties may arise, and to support you, and others, to be well and happy. In keeping with the Dalai Lama's advice: 'If you want others to be happy, practise compassion. If you want to be happy, practise compassion.'

Good luck, and many compassionate wishes!

Elaine and Chris

Resource bank

Throughout the workbook we have included a variety of exercises and information regarding websites that you may wish to use as an extra resource. In this section we have included blank templates, which you may find useful to work through.

In Chapter 18 (page 221) we used the following attention log to examine what you focused your attention on throughout the day.

Worksheet: Attention Log

Time and date	What was I doing?	Where was my attention focused?	How did my attention influence my feelings?	Was it possible to redirect attention if not focused on what I was doing?
Morning				
Afternoon				
Evening				
Night				

In Chapter 19 (page 234) we used the thought monitoring form to reflect on your thinking.

Worksheet: Threat–system–based thought monitoring form

Time of day	Type of thought (e.g. threat-based – worrying, ruminating, or reassuring)	Content of thought (e.g. about work, family, health, the future)	How did this thought affect my feelings? (e.g. anxious, angry, sad, happy)	How did I deal with the thought? (e.g. ignored it, tried to stop it, tried to push it out of mind, acted on it)
Morning				
Afternoon				
Evening				

In Chapter 19 (pages 243) we completed the Compassionate Thought Record. Here is a blank template that you could photocopy and use:

Worksheet 19.2: Compassionate Thought Record

Column 1 Triggering Events	Column 2 Unhelpful or Upsetting Thoughts and Images	Column 3 Feelings and Emotions	Column 4 Thought balancing – 'Helpful' or 'Balanced' Thoughts	Column 5 Understanding and Change in Feelings
What actually happened? What was the trigger?	*What am I thinking about others and their thoughts about me? What am I thinking about myself?*	*What are my main feelings and emotions?*	*What would I say to a friend?* *What compassionate alternatives might there be?* Empathy for my distress Compassionate attention Compassionate thinking Compassionate behaviour	*Write down any change in your feelings*

In Chapter 23 (pages 308) we completed a multiple self exercise. Here is an extra template.

Angry self	**Sad self**
Thoughts	Thoughts
Body	Body
Behaviour	Behaviour
Memory	Memory
Outcome	Outcome
Anxious self	**Compassionate self**
Thoughts	Thoughts
Body	Body
Behaviour	Behaviour
Memory	Memory
Outcome	Outcome

Index